CARDIOLOGY CLINICAL METHODS

CARDIOLOGY CLINICAL METHODS

V Jacob Jose
MD DM (card) FACC FCSI FIAE
Formerly, Professor and Head
Department of Cardiology
Christian Medical College and Hospital, Vellore
Tamil Nadu, India

S Ramakrishnan
MD DM (card) FACC
Professor
Department of Cardiology
All India Institute of Medical Sciences
New Delhi, India

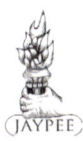

The Health Sciences Publisher
New Delhi | London | Panama

Jaypee Brothers Medical Publishers (P) Ltd

Headquarters

Jaypee Brothers Medical Publishers (P) Ltd
4838/24, Ansari Road, Daryaganj
New Delhi 110 002, India
Phone: +91-11-43574357
Fax: +91-11-43574314
Email: jaypee@jaypeebrothers.com

Overseas Offices

J.P. Medical Ltd
83 Victoria Street, London
SW1H 0HW (UK)
Phone: +44 20 3170 8910
Fax: +44 (0)20 3008 6180
Email: info@jpmedpub.com

Jaypee-Highlights Medical Publishers Inc
City of Knowledge, Bld. 235, 2nd Floor, Clayton
Panama City, Panama
Phone: +1 507-301-0496
Fax: +1 507-301-0499
Email: cservice@jphmedical.com

Jaypee Brothers Medical Publishers (P) Ltd
17/1-B Babar Road, Block-B, Shaymali
Mohammadpur, Dhaka-1207
Bangladesh
Mobile: +08801912003485
Email: jaypeedhaka@gmail.com

Jaypee Brothers Medical Publishers (P) Ltd
Bhotahity, Kathmandu
Nepal
Phone: +977-9741283608
Email: kathmandu@jaypeebrothers.com

Website: www.jaypeebrothers.com
Website: www.jaypeedigital.com

© 2017, Jaypee Brothers Medical Publishers

The views and opinions expressed in this book are solely those of the original contributor(s)/author(s) and do not necessarily represent those of editor(s) of the book.

All rights reserved. No part of this publication may be reproduced, stored or transmitted in any form or by any means, electronic, mechanical, photocopying, recording or otherwise, without the prior permission in writing of the publishers.

All brand names and product names used in this book are trade names, service marks, trademarks or registered trademarks of their respective owners. The publisher is not associated with any product or vendor mentioned in this book.

Medical knowledge and practice change constantly. This book is designed to provide accurate, authoritative information about the subject matter in question. However, readers are advised to check the most current information available on procedures included and check information from the manufacturer of each product to be administered, to verify the recommended dose, formula, method and duration of administration, adverse effects and contraindications. It is the responsibility of the practitioner to take all appropriate safety precautions. Neither the publisher nor the author(s)/editor(s) assume any liability for any injury and/or damage to persons or property arising from or related to use of material in this book.

This book is sold on the understanding that the publisher is not engaged in providing professional medical services. If such advice or services are required, the services of a competent medical professional should be sought.

Every effort has been made where necessary to contact holders of copyright to obtain permission to reproduce copyright material. If any have been inadvertently overlooked, the publisher will be pleased to make the necessary arrangements at the first opportunity.

Inquiries for bulk sales may be solicited at: jaypee@jaypeebrothers.com

Cardiology Clinical Methods

First Edition: **2017**

ISBN: 978-93-85999-45-1

Printed at

Dedicated to

My daughters
Riya Jose and
Nisha Jose

Contributors

Ashish Kumar MD DM (cardiology)
Cardiologist
Malabar Health Sciences
Calicut, Kerala, India

Bobby K John MD DM
Professor
Christian Medial College and Hospital
Vellore, Tamil Nadu, India

Devi MD (pediatrics) DM (cardiology)
Assistant Professor
Christian Medial College and Hospital
Vellore, Tamil Nadu, India

Oomen K George MD DM
Professor and Head
Department of Cardiology
Christian Medical College and Hospital
Vellore, Tamil Nadu, India

Parveen Kumar
Junior Consultant
Christian Medial College and Hospital
Vellore, Tamil Nadu, India

Preface

Clinical cardiology is slowly getting replaced by technology. Hand-carried echo machines and electronic stethoscopes have replaced the clinical skills that cardiologists learnt over a period of time by carefully examining the patient and listening to the heart sounds. However, they are still needed by Board exam-going students. In order to fill in the need for a textbook for Board examinations in cardiology, this book is written. We are sure the students taking up either DM in cardiology or DNB examinations will find it useful.

We are thankful to our colleagues, Dr Oomen George and Dr Bobby John for taking time to write several of the chapters in this book.

We also wish to thank Dr Parveen for editorial assistance. Special word of thanks to Dr Devi, our pediatric cardiologist, who was kind enough to go through some pediatric cardiology chapters.

We wish to express our colleagues in the department for their valuable inputs.

We are thankful to Ms Sabitha for her secretarial assistance.

We welcome critical remarks of the readers on this book so that the same can be followed for the improvement in the next edition.

V Jacob Jose
S Ramakrishnan

Contents

1 History Taking — 1
Dyspnea 1
Signals for the Sensation of Dyspnea 2
Orthopnea 2
Paroxysmal Nocturnal Dyspnea (PND) 3
Platypnea 3
Trepopnea 4
Orthostatic Dyspnea 4
Bendopnea 4
Causes of Dyspnea (Table 1) 4
Severity of Dyspnea Assessment 4
Indicators for Heart Failure as a Cause 6
Dyspnea and Valvular Heart Disease 6
Chest Pain 7
Angina 'Equivalents' 8
CCS Functional Classification for Angina 8
Syncope 9
Definition 9
Diagnostic Approach to Syncope 10
Scoring Systems for Syncope 10
Palpitations 10
Character of the Palpitations 11
Role of ECG for Clue to Diagnosis 11
Functional Classifications Used in Cardiology 11

2 Arterial Pulse — 12
Examination 12
Trisection of the pulse 12
Features of Arterial Pulse to be Examined 12
Rate 13
Rhythm 13
Character 14
Pulse in aortic regurgitation 15
C. Bisferiens Pulse 16
Pulsus Alternans 18
Pulsus Bigeminus 19
Pulsus Paradoxus 19
Volume of Pulse 21
Radiofemoral Delay 21
Condition of Vessel Wall 22

3 Blood Pressure — 23
White Coat Hypertension 23
Pseudohypertension 23
Orthostatic Hypotension 23

Methods of Measuring Arterial Blood Pressure 23
A. Direct method 23
B. Indirect Method 24
Korotkoff Sounds (KS) 24
Five phases 24
AHA Recommendations 24
Features Indicative of Secondary Causes 25
Guidelines for Measuring BP 25
Posture 25
Circumstances 25
Equipment 26
Technique 26
Valsalva Maneuver and Blood Pressure 26
Ambulatory BP Monitoring (ABPM) 27
Indications for ABPM 27
BP Thresholds—Definition 27
Goals in Hypertenson—JNC 2014 27

4 Jugular Venous Pulse 29
Determination of JVP 29
Technique of Examination 30
Methods to make JVP more obvious 30
Differences between the Venous and Arterial Pulsations 31
Normal Wave Pattern 31
A 31
B 31
a Wave 32
x Descent 32
c Wave 32
v Wave 32
y Descent 32
h Wave 32
Temporal Sequence with Cardiac Cycle 32
Normal Jugular Venous Pressure 33
Elevated Jugular Venous Pressure 33
Causes of Elevated JVP 33
Hepatojugular Reflux (Pasteur Rondot Maneuver) 33
A 34
B 34
Normal Response 34
HJR is Positive in 34
False-positive Hepatojugular Reflux 34
Alteration of "a" WAVE 35
x' Descent 36
Small x descent 36
Prominent x Descent 36
v WAVE 37
Prominent v waves 37

y Descent 37
Slow y descent 37
Deep y Descent 37
x versus y Descent 37
Kussmaul's Sign 38
Specific Cardiac Conditions 39
A. Atrial Septal Defect 39
B. Tricuspid Regurgitation 39
C. Constrictive Pericarditis 39
D. Eisenmenger Syndrome 40
E. Jugular Venous Wave Forms in Cyanotic Heart Disease 40

5 Precordial Examination—Palpation 41

Apex Beat 42
Definition 42
Mechanism 42
Point of Maximal Impulse (PMI) 45
Character of Apical Impulse 45
Sustained Apical Impulse 45
Hyperdynamic Apical Impulse 46
Hypokinetic Impulse 46
Ectopic Impulse 47
Parasternal Lift 48
Causes of Parasternal Lift 49
Dressler's Grading of Parasternal lift 50
Epigastric Impulse 50
PA Impulse 50
AORTIC Impulse 50
Thrills 51
Palpable Sounds 52

6 First Heart Sound 54

First Heart Sound 54
Components of First Heart Sound 54
Theories of Generation of First Heart Sound 54
Intensity of S1 55
Loud First Heart Sound 56
Causes of Loud S1 56
Mitral Stenosis 56
Soft First Heart Sound 56
Causes of Soft S1 56
Split S1 57
Reverse Splitting of S1 57
Hemodynamic Correlation of S1 57

7 Second Heart Sound 58

Theories of Generation of Second Heart Sound 58
Hang Out Interval 58
Abnormalities of S2 Intensity 58
Increased Intensity of P2 59

Soft P2 59
Splitting of S2 59
Mechanism of Splitting 59
Types of S2 Splitting 60
Wide Split S2 (Also Called as Persistent Split) 60
Other Causes 61
Fixed Splitting 61
Reversed or Paradoxical Splitting 61
Type I Paradoxical Splitting (The Most common) 61
Type II Paradoxical Splitting 62
Type III Paradoxical Splitting 62
Pseudoparadoxical Splitting 63
Narrow Physiologic Splitting 63
Single S2 63
II. Fusion of a2 and p2 63
III. Apparently Single S2 (Due to Inaudibility of P2) 64

8   Third Heart Sound — 65

Mechanism of Production of Third Heart Sound 65
Impact Theory (Most Accepted) 65
Ventricular Theory by Leatham 65
Valvular Theory 65
Clinical 66
Causes of Lv S3 67
Causes of Rv S3 67
Differentiation of S3 and Opening Snap 67

9   Fourth Heart Sound — 68

Mechanism of Production 68
Left Ventricular S4 68
Right Ventricular S4 68
Temporal Sequence 69
Fourth Heart Sound in Disease Conditions 69
1. *Atrioventricular Block 69*
2. *Coronary Artery Disease 69*
3. *Cardiomyopathy 70*
4. *Systemic Hypertension 70*
5. *Aortic Valve Disease 70*
6. *Age 70*
7. *Pulmonary Hypertension 70*
8. *Pulmonary Stenosis 70*
9. *Bernheim Phenomenon 70*
10. *Other Conditions 70*

Differentiation of M1–T1 From S4–S1 70
Summation Gallop 71

10 Systolic and Diastolic Sounds — 72

Ejection Clicks 72
Early Systolic Sounds 72
Mechanism of Production 72
Ejection Sounds and Phases of Respiration 72

Aortic Ejection Sound 73
Pulmonary Ejection Click 73
Pulmonary ES in Valvular PS 74
Pulmonary ES in PH or IDPA 74
Non-Ejction Clicks 74
Mitral Valve Prolapse 74
Opening Snap 75
S2 - OS interval 76
S2-OS Interval and Its Relationship to the Severity of Mitral Stenosis 77
Causes of Soft OS in Mitral Stenosis 77
Differentiation Of S3 and Opening Snap 77
Pericardial Knock 77
Prosthetic Valve Sounds 78

11 Diastolic Murmurs 79

Classification 79
Mechanism 79
Early Diastolic Murmurs 80
Aortic Regurgitation 80
Musical Diastolic Murmur 81
Mid-Diastolic Murmur (MDM) 83
Mitral Stenosis 83
Tricuspid Stenosis 85
Rytand Murmur 86
Carey Coombs Murmur 86
Flow Murmur 86
Pulmonary Regurgitation 87
Late Diastolic or Presystolic Murmurs 87
Mitral Stenosis 87
Tricuspid Stenosis 88
Complete Heart Block 88
Austin Flint Murmur 88
Bioprosthetic Valve 89

12 Continuous Murmurs 90

Mechanisms of Continuous Murmurs [Myer's Classification (1975)] 90
Patent Ductus Arteriosus (Machinery Murmur or Gibsons Murmur) 91
Aortopulmonary Window 92
Congenital Coronary Arterial Fistula 92
General Principles 92
Rupture of Sinus Valsalva Aneurysm 93
RSOV into RA 93
RSOV into RV 93
Anomalous Origin of Left Coronary Artery from the Pulmonary Artery (Bland White Garland Syndrome) 94
Congenital Pulmonary AV Fistula 94

Acquired Arteriovenous Fistula 94
Lutembacher Syndrome 94
Murmurs Occurring in Constricted Arteries 95
Continuous Murmur Arising from Collaterals between Systemic and Pulmonary Arteries 95
Venous Hum 95
Two Mechanisms Proposed for Venous Hum 96
Continuous Murmur with Cyanosis 96

13. Rheumatic Fever   97

Group A Beta Hemolytic Streptococci - GABHS 97
Prevalence of Rheumatic Heart Disease in India 97
Age of RF 98
Criteria for Diagnosis 98
Exceptions to Jones Criteria 99
Arthritis 99
Jaccoud's arthritis 100
Carditis 100
Valve Involvement in Acute Rheumatic Fever 101
Valve Combinations in Indian Data for Chronic RHD (IHJ 2014: 320- 326) 101
Carditis—Role of Echo 101
Chorea 103
Signs 103
Duration 104
Sequelae 104
Preceding Streptococcal Infection within Last 45 Days—Mandatory Criteria 104
Clinical Course 105
Treatment 105
Rheumatic Fever Recurrence Rates Using Drugs 107
Treatment of Chorea 107

14. Aortic Stenosis   110

Hemodynamics 110
Etiology of Valvar AS 111
Progression 112
History 112
Reasons for Angina 113
Physical findings 114
Chest X-ray 115
ECG 115
Echo Assessment of AS 115
Coronary Angiography 115
Natural History 116
Surgery 118
Indications for Surgery ACC/AHA 2014[10] 118
Bicuspid Valve and Aortic Root Surgery (JACC Dec 4, 2015) 118

Statins and Aortic Stenosis Progression 118
Low Flow Low Gradient As 119
Low Dose Dobutamine Echo Test 119
Aortic Stenosis with Regurgitation 119
Transcatheter Aortic Valve Replacement – TAVI 120
Indications for Transcatheter AVR – 2014 AHA/ACC Guidelines 120

15 Aortic Regurgitation 122
Etiology 122
Pathophysiology 122
LV remodeling 122
Clinical 123
Arterial Pulse 123
Peripheral Signs 124
Precordial Examination 125
Auscultation 125
Mechanism 126
Chest X-Ray 126
ECG 126
Natural History 128
Treatment 128
Vasodilators 128
Indications for Surgery in Severe AR 129
Recommendations for Angiogram in Severe AR: 129

16 Mitral Stenosis 130
Etiology 130
Hemodynamics 130
Valve Area and Gradients 131
Features of LA Pressure Tracing 131
Pulmonary Hypertension 131
Atrial fibrillation 131
History 131
Auscultation 133
Loud First Heart Sound 133
Opening Snap 133
Mid Diastolic Murmur 134
Presystolic Murmur (PSM) 135
Chest X-ray 135
ECG 136
Natural History 136
Management 136
PTMC/BMV Indications 136
Restenosis after PTMC 137
Effect of PTMC and Atrial Fibrillation 137
20 year Results of PTMC 137
Juvenile MS 138
ECHO Approach to Mitral Stenosis 138
Left Atrial Clot 138

17. Mitral Regurgitation — 140

Etiology 140
Types of MR 140
Clinical Examination 140
Precordial Examination 140
Heart Sounds 140
MR Murmur 141
Maneuvers 142
Thrill 142
ECHO Grading of Severity 143
Natural History 143
Surgery 144
Mitral Valve Repair 145
Predictors of Recurrent Functional MR after Annuloplasty 145
Medical Treatment for Primary MR 145

18. Prosthetic Valve — 147

Case Scenario 147
Types of Valves 147
Mechanical 147
Tissue 147
Auscultation 148
Anticoagulation 148
Mechanical Valves 148
Tissue Valves 148
Risk of Bleeding with Warfarin 149
Mechanical or Tissue Valve 149
Randomized Studies on Mechanical versus Tissue Valves 149
Aortic Homograft 149
Investigations 149
Complications 151
2. Embolism 152
3. Endocarditis (PVE) 152
4. Valve Dysfunction 152
Porcine versus Pericardial Valve 153
5. Hemolysis 153
Excessive Anticoagulation 153
Bridging Therapy 154
Coronary Angiogram before Valve Surgery 155
Heart Failure after Valve Replacement 155
AFIB Ablation During Mitral Valve Replacement 155
Trans Catheter Aortic Valve Replacement 155
Contraindications 156
Complications 156
Limitations between Medtronic and Edwards Sapien Valves 156

19 Hypertrophic Cardiomyopathy — 158

Prevalence 158
Pathogenesis 158
Myocardial Fibrosis 159
Causes of Myocardial Ischemia 159
Mitral Regurgitation in HCM 159
Genes Associated with HCM 159
Family Screening by Echo or CMR (JACC July 2012) 160
Clinical Features—Obstructive Cardiomyopathy 160
Mid-ventricular Obstruction 161
Valsalva and HCM 162
Alcohol and Obstructive HCM 162
Yamaguchi's Apical HCM 163
ECG Features of HCM 163
ECHO 163
Electrophysiologic Studies 165
Hemodynamics 165
Natural History 165
Sudden Death 165
SCD Risk Modifiers 166
Gene Mutations and Survival 166
SCD Risk Calculation Formula 166
TMT Testing in HCM 167
Treatment 167
Drug Therapy 167
Surgery—Myectomy/Morrow procedure 168
Alcohol Septal Ablation (PTSMA) 168
Effects of PTSMA on the Conduction System 168
Predictors for Complete Heart Block 168
Complications of PTSMA 169
PTSMA Concerns 169
Indications 169
Technique 169
Survival—Long Term Results for PTSMA 170
Radiofrequency Septal Ablation for HCM 170
PTSMA versus Surgical Myectomy 170
PTSMA versus Myectomy—Survival Differences 170
Differential Diagnosis of HCM 170
HCM and Pregnancy 172

20 Constrictive Pericorditis — 174

Constrictive Pericarditis 174
Syndromes of Constrictive Pericarditis 174
Pathoanatomical Forms 174
Etiology 175
Pathophysiology 175
Clinical Signs of Constrictive Pericarditis 175

ECG Changes 175
Chest X-ray 175
Echo Signs *176*
Hemodynamic Criteria 177
Role of Cardiac MRI *177*
Pericardectomy 177

21 Aortoarteritis 178
Historical Perspective 178
Etiopathogenesis 178
Classification 179
I. Proposed by Ueno et al. and Later Modified by Lupi Herrera 179
II. Takayasu Conference 1994 180
Clinical Features 180
Criteria for Diagnosis 181
Natural History 184
Complications 184
Uyama and Asayama Classification of Retinopathy 185
Assessment of Disease Activity 185
Investigations 186
Treatment 187
Medical treatment 187
Indications for Revascularization 188
Prognosis 188
Predictors of an Acute Event 188
Results of Intervention 188
Coarctation of Aorta 189
Physical Appearance 189
Turner's syndrome 189
Signs 189
Chest X-Ray 190
Natural History 191
Treatment 191

22 Approach to Congenital Heart Disease 192
Genetic Aspects of Congenital Heart Disease 192
Consanguinity 192
Folic Acid and Congenital Treat Disease 192
Clinical Features of CHD 193
Role of Hyperoxia Test 196
Teratogens 196
Bedside Approach to Cyanotic Congenital Heart Disease 197
Key Points on Genetic Aspects 199

23 Eisenmenger Syndrome 200
Definition 200
ES Starts at Infancy in Age at Presentation of ES 200
Size of the Defect and ES 200
Ventricle Overload in ES 200
Prevalence of PH with CHD 200

Clinical Classification of Congenital Heart Disease 201
Symptoms 201
Signs 202
ECG 202
Differences Between the Groups 202
Morphometric Grading 203
Alveloar Arterial Ratio 203
Simple Methods to Decide on Operability 204
Treatment 204
Survival 207
Survival of Treatment Naïve Patients with ES 207
Suggested Treatment Algorithm for ES 207

24 Tetralogy of Fallot or Ventricular Septal Defect Plus Pulmonary Stenosis 209

Anatomy 209
Spectrum of TOF Anatomy 209
Embryology 209
Prevalence 209
Environmental Factors 210
Association with Genetic Disorders 210
Role of Karyotyping 210
Facial Features 211
Types of VSD 211
Morphologic Categories of RVOT Obstruction 211
Haffman's Variant 212
Papillary Muscles of RV 212
Coronary Anomalies 212
Major Associated Cardiac Defects 212
Minor Associated Anomalies 212
Clinical Features 212
Pink Tets/TET 212
Cyanosis 212
Squatting 213
Spell/Hypoxic Spell 213
Recurrent Respiratory Tract Infections 214
Clubbing 214
Jugular Venous Pulse 214
Precordial Palpation 214
Auscultation 214
Features of Adult TOF 215
Chest X-Ray 215
ECG 216
ECG axis 216
Oxymetry 217
Angiogram 217
Complications of TOF 217
Infective Endocarditis 217
Differential Diagnosis 217
Within the VSD + PS Physiology 217

Differences between VSD + PS versus PS with ASD 218
Treatment of A Spell 218
Catheter Interventions in TOF 219
Surgery 219
Primary Repair versus Palliation 219
Annular Patch 219
Assessment of the Adequacy of PA Size 220
Types of Shunts 220
BT Shunt History 221
Central Shunt 221
Watterson Shunt 222
Glenn Shunt 222
Repaired TOF 222
Pulmonary Valve Replacement 223
Summary Indications for PVR 224
Results of PVR 224
Methods Used for PVR 225

25. Pulmonary Atresia with VSD 227
Incidence 227
Morphology 227
Environmental and Genetic factors 227
Embryology 227
Pathology 228
Collateral Anatomy in PA VSD 229
Collateral Artery Supply Differences 229
Differences between Ductus and MAPCA 229
Classification 230
Congenital Heart Surgery and Database Project based on PA anatomy 230
Somerville Classification 230
Clinical 230
Chest X-Ray 230
Multidetector computed tomography 230
Differential Diagnosis 230
Natural History 231
Management 231
Palliative Surgery 231
Intracardiac Repair 232
Treatment Based on Pulmonary Circulation 232
Results of Surgery 233

26. Chest X-Ray 235
AP versus PA—Heart Size 235
Assessing Inspiration 235
Penetration 236
Assessing heart size 236
Left Atrium Enlargement 236
Causes of Double Density 237

Right Atrium 237
Left Ventricle 237
PA View 238
Lateral View 238
Right Ventricle 238
Lateral View 238
PA View 238
Pulmonary Blood Flow 238
Increased Pulmonary Vascularity 238
Pulmonary Artery Hypertension 239
Pulmonary Artery Stenosis 239
Decreased Pulmonary Blood Flow 239
Congestive Cardiac Failure 239
Grading of Pulmonary Venous Hypertension 240
Grading of PVH and PCW 240
Pleural Effusion in Heart Failure 241

27. ECG Criterias 242

Left Atrial Enlargement 242
Right Atrial Enlargement 242
Biatrial Enlargement 242
Right Ventricular Hypertrophy 243
Buttler and Legget Criteria for RVH 243
Left Ventricular Hypertrophy: Voltage Criteria 243
Left Ventricular Hypertrophy—Romhilt-Estes Point Score System 243
Paediatric Criteria for Left Ventricular Hypertrophy (Age-Related) 244
Paediatric Criteria for Right Ventricular Hypertrophy (Age-Related) 244
Stepwise Criteria Favoring Ventricular Tachycardia 244

Index 247

CHAPTER 1

History Taking

V Jacob Jose

CHAPTER OUTLINE

- Dyspnea
- Chest Pain
- Syncope
- Functional Classifications used in Cardiology

Four symptoms need to be covered in the history and they are as follows:
1. Dyspnea
2. Chest pain
3. Syncope
4. Palpitations

DYSPNEA

Definition

Dyspnea is defined as an "abnormally uncomfortable awareness of breathing." The word dyspnea is derived from Greek, meaning dys-difficult and pnoia – breathing.

The American Thoracic Society has defined Dyspnea as "subjective experience of breathing discomfort that consists of qualitatively distinct sensations that vary in intensity."

Chronic dyspnea is defined as dyspnea lasting longer than one month.

Qualitative descriptors
- Chest tightness: Bronchospasm, interstitial edema, myocardial ischemia
- Increased work of breathing: COPD
- Air Hunger: CHF, Pulmonary embolism
- Cannot get deep breath: Hyperinflation
- Heavy breathing: Deconditioning.

Mechanism of Dyspnea (Chest 2010; 138: 1196 – 1201)

Hypothetical Model (Gillette and Schwartstein)

- Afferents reach the sensory cortex
- The motor cortex sends neural messages to ventilator muscles and also a discharge to sensory cortex

- When the feedforward and feedback do not match, an error signal is generated and the intensity of dyspnea increases.

Signals for the Sensation of Dyspnea

Afferent information from reflex stimulation of the peripheral sensors (chemoreceptors or vagal C fibers) is processed in the Limbic system and sensorimotor cortex and increased neural output to respiratory muscles. A perturbation in the ventilatory response due to increased mechanical load or weakness or paralysis generates afferent information from vagal receptors in the lungs and possibly mechanoreceptors in the respiratory muscles to the sensorimotor cortex and results in the sensation of dyspnea.

It has been shown that vagal C fibers from the jugular ganglion (**jugular C fibers**) are associated with larger airways. Deeper C fibers in the lungs are associated with nodose ganglia (**nodose C fibers**). Nodose fibers are stimulated by adenosine. Experiments have shown that IV adenosine can cause dyspnea but no cough and this can be blocked by theophylline and also by inhaled lidocaine (Fig. 1).

Orthopnea

- Dyspnea in supine posture, relieved by sitting up.
- This is due to increased venous return in supine posture leads to more pulmonary congestion

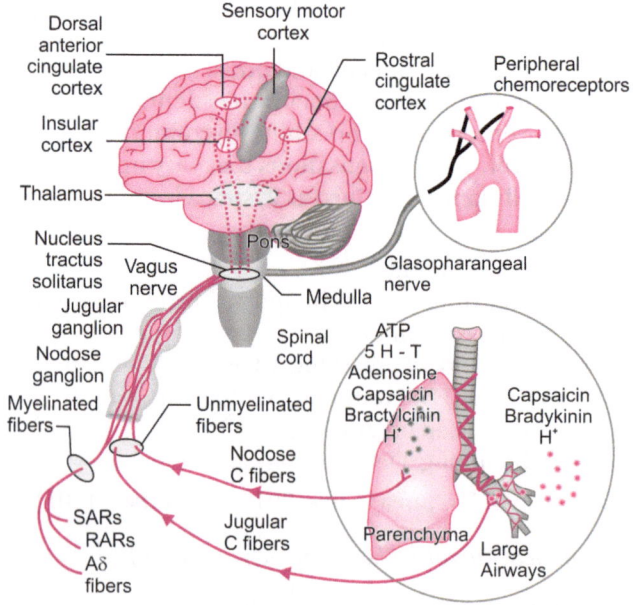

Figure 1 Pathway for dyspnea (Adapted from Chest November 2010)

- Also any respiratory distress, there is a mechanical advantage on sitting up for the respiratory muscles so that patient feels better
- Causes of orthopnea:
  - Left heart failure
  - COPD
  - Large ascites
  - Bilateral diaphragmatic paralysis
  - Any severe right heart failure.

Paroxysmal Nocturnal Dyspnea (PND)

- In this form of dyspnea, breathing difficulty occurs 2-6 hours after sleep, especially in the early morning hours.
- This is due to interstitial edema of the lung
- The suggested mechanism is that, there is decreased sympathetic drive during sleep decreases the functional capacity after ventricle. In addition increased absorption of edema fluid results in overfilling of the lungs
- Conditions that can mimic PND are:
  - Bronchial Asthma
  - Sleep apnea with arousal
  - Postnasal discharge with cough
  - Nocturnal angina with dyspnea equivalent.

Platypnea

This type of dyspnea occurs in sitting posture. This can occur in left atrial myxoma or with ball valve thrombus of left atrium.

Platypnoea-orthodeoxia is an uncommon syndrome of dyspnea induced by **upright posture**, with associated **arterial hypoxemia**, which is subsequently relieved by recumbency. The syndrome occurs when there is right to left shunting of blood, usually via an interatrial communication, in the presence of normal pulmonary artery pressure. This is an unusual situation given that most cases of significant right to left intracardiac shunting of blood are associated with increased right-sided cardiac pressures.

Various theories have been advanced to explain why patients with a patent foramen ovale may develop this syndrome.
1. Preferential blood flow directed towards the atrial septum, which can be accentuated by altered intracardiac anatomical relations.
2. Unequal diastolic compliance between the right and left sides of the heart, and transient right to left pressure gradients associated with respiratory maneuvers, all of which can result in significant right to left shunting in the upright position.

The treatment of choice is to close the interatrial communication.

Trepopnea

This type of dyspnea occurs in lateral decubitus. The causes are pleural effusion or large mass lesions of lung.

Orthostatic Dyspnea

Orthostatic dyspnea is thought to reflect ventilation-perfusion mismatch due to inadequate perfusion of ventilated lung apices. It can even be orthostatic angina (attributed to impaired myocardial perfusion even with normal coronary arteries.

Bendopnea (JACC heart failure Feb 2014)

Definition

Shortness of breath, specifically when bending forward, such as when putting on their shoes or socks.

Mechanism
During bending, increased intrathoracic pressure leads to a further increase in ventricular filling pressures, and subjects with bendopnea (who start with higher filling pressures) are more likely to reach a threshold pressure necessary to induce shortness of breath. It is likely caused by elevation in the left-sided filling pressure, or pulmonary capillary wedge pressure (PCWP), as has been demonstrated with other manifestations of shortness of breath in patients with heart failure.

Causes of Dyspnea (Table 1)

Dyspnea can be classified into acute dyspnea at rest or chronic breathlessness on exertion (BOE).

Severity of Dyspnea Assessment

For practical purposes, we follow the New York Heart Association (NYHA), functional classification for grading the severity of dyspnea which is given in the Table 2A and B. There

Table 1
Causes of dyspnea

System	Acute dyspnea at rest	Chronic exertional dyspnea
Cardio-vascular system	Acute pulmonary edema Pulmonary embolism Major congenital heart disease	Chronic cardiac failure Chronic pulmonary thromboembolism Congenital heart disease
Respiratory system	Acute severe asthma Acute COPD Pneumothorax Pneumonia	COPD Chronic asthma Bronchial carcinoma Interstitial lung disease

Contd...

Contd...

System	Acute dyspnea at rest	Chronic exertional dyspnea
	Acute respiratory distress syndrome Inhaled foreign body Lobar collapse Laryngeal oedema (e.g. anaphylaxis)	Lymphatic carcinomatosis (may cause intolerable dyspnoea) Large pleural effusion(s)
Others	Metabolic acidosis Hysterical / Psychogenic hyperventilation	Severe anemia

Table 2A
NYHA functional classification

1	Patients with cardiac disease but without resulting limitations of physical activity. Ordinarily physical activity does not cause undue fatigue, palpitation, dyspnea, or anginal pain
2	Patients with cardiac disease resulting in slight limitation of physical activity. They are comfortable at rest. Ordinarily physical activity results in fatigue, palpitation, dyspnea, or anginal pain
3	Patients with cardiac disease resulting in marked limitation of physical activity. They are comfortable at rest. Less than ordinary physical activity causes fatigue, palpitation, dyspnea, or anginal pain
4	Patients with cardiac disease resulting in inability to carry on any physical activity without discomfort. Symptoms of cardiac insufficiency or of the angina syndrome may be present even at rest. If any physical activity is undertaken, discomfort is increased.

Table 2B
NYHA classification

6th edition 1964	9th edition 1994
Etiology	Functional
Anatomy	Objective
Physiology	
Functional	
Therapeutic	

are others, such as specific activity scale American Thoracic Society (ATS) and Medical Research Council (MRC) as well.

The limitations of NYHA classification:
1. Subjective
2. Reproducibility is low

Table 3
Goldman specific activity scale

1	Patients can perform to completion any activity requiring 7 METs or more.
2	Patients can perform to completion any activity requiring 5 METs but not 7 METs
3	Patients can perform to completion any activity requiring 2 METs but not 5 METs
4	Patients cannot or do not perform to completion activities requiring 2 METs or more

Hence a good way of precisely quantifying the severity of dyspnea has been put forward in the specific activity scale which is given Table 3.

The original NYHA classification includes five components, but we use only the functional component.

Indicators for Heart Failure as a Cause

- Third heart sound – Likelihood ratio – 24
- Displaced apical impulse – LR 16.5
- Jugular venous distension – LR 8.5
- If all three are there, it is virtually diagnostic of heart failure.

Dyspnea and Valvular Heart Disease

- **Mitral Stenosis:** This is the main symptom of MS. It is due to pulmonary venous hypertension. As a rule, if patient has dyspnea + PND for more than 5 years, then MS is most likely underlying condition. The severity of dyspnea also correlates well with 10 year survival. NYHA class 2 persons survival for 10 years is only 50% whereas if class 4, it is only 20% from studies done in the prevalvotomy era.
- **Mitral Regurgitation:** Dyspnea is a late symptom of MR except in acute MR. It is due to pulmonary venous hypertension. The reasons for PVH are:
  - Left ventricle failure
  - MR with noncompliant left atrium
  - Associated mitral stenosis
  - Arrhythmias' with fast heart rate, such as atrial fibrillation
- **Aortic Stenosis:** Dyspnea is a late symptom and survival is only about 1.5 year after the onset of this symptom. If the duration of dyspnea is more than 5 years with aortic stenosis, then suspect associated mitral valve disease. The reasons for dyspnea in AS is multifactorial:
  - LV systolic dysfunction
  - LV diastolic dysfunction due to LVH
  - Associated mitral valve disease
  - Associated coronary artery disease

- **Aortic Regurgitation:** Dyspnea occurs very late in the course of AR. It is also slow to progress in AR. Some patients with AR feel better on walking and this is due to the fact that on walking the heart rate increases, the duration of diastole comes down and the volume of regurgitation decreases. Exercise-induced peripheral vasodilatation may also contribute to the reduction of AR.

CHEST PAIN

Chest pain can be classified into acute, severe on going chest pain and episodic chest pain. The later form is further classified into three types, based on three features.
- Typical chest pain
- Atypical chest pain
- Noncardiac chest pain.

Typical chest pain (PQR)
- **P**recipitated by exertion or emotional stress
- **Q**uality: Pressure/Heaviness
- **R**elieved by rest or nitroglycerin.

Atypical
Meets only two of the three above characteristics.

Noncardiac chest pain
Meets only one of the angina characteristics (Table 4A and B).

Table 4A

Various terminologies for angina

Stable angina	A predictable pattern regarding frequency and precipitating factors (sustained over > 2 months)
New onset	Recently developed angina (within the previous 1 to 3 months)
Primary angina	Angina at rest with obvious precipitating cause. If primary angina develops with exercise, the level at which it occurs in inconsistent. A synonym for this type of angina is "variable threshold" angina
Secondary angina	Typical exertional angina associated with specific and usually predictable forms and levels of physical activity
Mixed angina	Composite pattern of primary and secondary angina
Emotional angina	Angina with specific psychological factors that precipitate symptoms
Nocturnal angina	Angina that awakens and is sometimes associated with dreaming or sleep apnea
Angina decubitus	Angina that occurs shortly after adopting the recumbent posture. May coexist with nocturnal angina

Contd...

Contd...

Status anginosus	Frequent, recurrent, sustained angina refractory to usual treatment
Walk-through angina	Angina with effort that disappears gradually during activity that is sustained (although usually at reduced intensity) and after which improved exercise tolerance results
Second-wind angina	A brief rest after an initial attack results in a markedly improved threshold free from angina. A synonym is "warm-up" angina
Caudal angina	Symptoms occurring in the scalp or head referred pain
Silent angina	Objective manifestations of ischemia without symptoms
Crescendo angina	Synonym is "accelerated" angina. Change in the pattern of angina such that it comes on more easily, lasts longer, or is more frequent

Table 4B

Points in history for chest pain

1	Site of pain: Center, side of chest
2	Radiation: To jaw, to left arm, right arm
3	Duration of pain: In minutes/continuous/episodic
4	Precipitating factor: Related to effort, food
5	Relieving factors: Rest/nitro relief
6	Associated symptoms: Sweating, breathing difficulty

Angina 'Equivalents'

1. Dyspnea
2. Jaw or neck discomfort
3. Shoulder or elbow pain
4. Epigastric discomfort
5. Interscapular discomfort

Blockpnea (Chevalier, American Heart Journal 1961; 73: 579 – 581)

This term was put forward by **Gallavardin** in the year 1933, for the feeling of blocked respiration or suffocation while walking. This is actually the **dyspnea equivalent**.

CCS Functional Classification for Angina

- Class 1: Ordinary physical activity, such as walking or climbing stairs does not cause angina. Angina occurs **at strenuous or rapid or prolonged exertion** at work or recreation.
- Class 2: Slight limitation of physical activity. Walking **more than 2 blocks** or one flight of ordinary stairs at normal pace and in normal conditions.

- Class 3: **Walking one or 2 blocks** and climbing more than one flight of ordinary stairs in normal conditions
- Class 4: Inability to carry on any physical activity without discomfort – anginal syndrome may be present at rest.

SYNCOPE

(Greek word: syn = with; koptein = to cut or to interrupt)

Definition

Syncope is a transient loss of consciousness (T-LOC) due to transient global cerebral hypoperfusion characterized by **rapid onset, short duration, and spontaneous recovery**

Near syncope is defined as transient loss of postural tone. The underlying mechanism of syncope is transient global cerebral hypoperfusion.

Usual duration of syncope is not more than **20 seconds** on an average (Table 5).

History taking: The following **five** points need to be taken in history.

1. **Preceding events:** From the history, you must ask whether syncope happened after prolonged standing or seeing some unusual sight, such as an accident, or turning the head, etc.

Table 5

Differentiating features of seizure versus syncope

		Seizure	Syncope
1	Preceding events	None	Standing for a long time. Seeing blood
2	Type of onset	Sudden	Gradual
3	Position at onset	Any	Standing may be (Can occur supine)
4	Aura	+	-
5	Facial – Cyanosis	+	-
6	Tongue biting	+	-
7	Incontinence of Urine	+	+ / -
8	Duration of tonic and clonic movements	> 30 sec	Less than 15 seconds
9	Post ictal amnesia	+	
10	Post ictal confusion	Less than 30 seconds	Longer
11	Post ictal headache	+	
12	Rapid recovery	Minutes to hours	Less than 5 min

2. **Type on onset:** The onset is sudden in arrhythmia and in seizures. It is gradual in vasovagal syndrome.
3. **Position at onset:** This history is important because arrhythmia can happen in any position. However, vasovagal syncope occurs on standing for a long time.
4. **Postsyncopal clearing:** Clearing of consciousness is gradual and takes a long time in seizures where as it is very brief in cardiac reasons.
5. **Associated events:** Tongue biting, urinary incontinence are common with seizures.
   - **The single most powerful factor is postictal confusion** as observed by an eyewitness. Reorientation is usually immediate in syncope and **does not exceed 30 seconds** even after extended attacks. (Annals of Internal Medicine, 1988; 108: 791- 796).
   - Incontinence and head injury are common in both conditions. (Jour of Royal Society of Med July 1996)

Diagnostic Approach to Syncope

- Is it vertigo?
- Is it loss of balance?
- Light headed? To Transient Loss of Consciousness – T-LOC
- Seizure?

Scoring Systems for Syncope

There are many scoring systems for syncope. One of them is **EGSYS score**.(A. Del Roso, Heart 2008; 94: 1620) six variables are included and point weightage score is given. A score of 3 or more needs a cardiologist evaluation. This calculation application is available in the smart phone systems.
- Palpitations preceding syncope – 4
- Heart disease or abnormal ECG – 3
- Syncope during effort – 3
- Syncope while supine – 2
- Precipitating factors – minus 1
- Autonomic prodromes – minus 1.

Palpitations

Palpitations can be defined as uncomfortable awareness of heart beats.

History should include the following:
- Character of the palpitations
- Onset and offset
- Precipitating factors
- Associated symptoms
- Frequency or incidence.

Character of the Palpitations (Lancet May 1993; 1254)

- Rapid, regular and frog positive: AV nodal tachycardia
- Rapid regular and frog negative: AVRT or AT or VT
- Rapid and irregular – AFib
- Slow and regular and frog positive: VPC
- Slow, regular and frog negative: Any VPC.

During AV nodal re-entrant tachycardia, atria and ventricles contract simultaneously, causing pronounced reflux of blood into the superior vena cava and the feeling of neck pulsations. Because of this patient may look like frog under these circumstances and this is called as **frog positive by Brugada.** This is also called **as pounding in the neck.**

Role of ECG for Clue to Diagnosis (NEJM May 1998: 338: 1369)

1. Short PR: Pre-excitation
2. P mitrale or frequent APC: AFib
3. VPC's, LBBB with positive axis: RVOT ventricular tachycardia
4. VPC's with RBBB with negative axis: Idiopathic VT – LV type
5. Q waves: Old MI
6. Complete AV block
7. Long QT: polymorphic VT
8. Inverted T in v1 and Epsilon wave: ARVD

FUNCTIONAL CLASSIFICATIONS USED IN CARDIOLOGY

1. NYHA for Dyspnea
2. CCS for Angina
3. WHO classification in Pulmonary Hypertension
4. **EHRA** for AFib

CHAPTER 2

Arterial Pulse

Oomen K George, Bobby John

CHAPTER OUTLINE

- Definition
- Examination
- Rate
- Rhythm
- Character
- Volume of Pulse
- Radiofemoral Delay
- Condition of Vessel Wall

DEFINITION

Pulse is a pressure wave originating in the aorta due to ejection of blood during left ventricular systole and the wave travels along the arterial wall at a rate much faster than the actual column of blood (Pulse wave velocity is 5 m/s. Velocity of intraluminal blood is 40–50 cm/s).

EXAMINATION

Palpation of arteries: Press with the examining fingers until maximum pulse is sensed. Pulse is felt as changing displacement superimposed on the baseline displacement produced by compressing the artery. The index finger is the best finger to feel the pulse.

Scale for comparing the pulse

0 : Absent pulse
1+ : Present but diminished pulse
2+ : Average normal pulse
3+ : Moderately increased
4+ : Markedly increased pulse.

Trisection of the Pulse

Varying decrease of pressure should be applied with the thumb or forefinger until the maximum pulse is sensed while concentrating on the sharpness of the upstroke, systolic peak, and diastolic slope of the arterial pulse.

FEATURES OF ARTERIAL PULSE TO BE EXAMINED

1. Rate
2. Rhythm

3. Character
4. Volume
6. Vessel wall thickness
7. Peripheral pulses
8. Radiofemoral delay

RATE

The resting heart rate shows considerable variation ranging between 50 and 120 beats/min. Rate should be counted for at least 30 seconds. When rhythm is irregular, count for 60s.

Pulse deficit: The rate of palpable arterial pulse is slower than the rate of ventricular contraction, e.g. atrial fibrillation or marked pulsus alternans. Pulse deficit is identified by comparing the rate of arterial pulse (palpable) with the heart rate judged by simultaneous precordial auscultation. In order to observe the pulse deficit it is better to have two persons simultaneously examine the patients; one person will count the heart rate using the stethoscope; the second person will count the pulse rate from the radial artery. The deficit is said to be significant if the difference between heart rate and the pulse rate is **more than 10**. If a second observer is not available then you may first count the heart rate by auscultation and then subsequently count the pulse rate using the radial artery (Table 1).

RHYTHM

This can be regular or irregular. If irregular observe whether irregularity has a recurring pattern or completely irregular or whether an otherwise regular rhythm is occasionally interrupted by some slight irregularity.

Equality of Pulses

Unequal carotid pulsations occur in the following:
1. Carotid atherosclerosis.
2. Takayasu's disease.
3. Aortic arch aneurysm.

Table 1
Causes of irregular and regular pulse

Irregularly irregular	Regular
Sinus Arrhythmia	Fixed heart block
Atrial fibrillation	Ventricular tachycardia
VPCs or SVPCs	Complete heart block
Varying heart block	Normal
PAT with Block	
Atrial flutter with varying block	

4. Aortic dissection.
5. Supravalvular AS.

Unequal upper extremity pulses:
1. Supravalvular AS.
2. Coarctation of aorta.
3. Anomalous origin or aberrant path of major vessels.
4. Cervical rib.
5. Arterial embolus/thrombosis.

CHARACTER

The normal pulse has a smooth rapid upstroke, (the ascending limb), smooth dome shaped summit and a down stroke, less rapid than the upstroke. The volume and contour of the arterial pulse are determined by a combination of factors, including the LV stroke volume, ejection velocity, the relative compliance and capacity of the arterial system and the pressure waves that result from the antegrade flow of blood and reflection of the arterial pressure pulse returning from the peripheral circulation.

Graphic recording of arterial pulse show two positive deflections in systole, first being the percussion wave and second the *tidal wave*. Percussion wave represents the arrival of impulse generated by LV ejection, tidal wave represent its echo from the upper part of the body and the third wave; dicrotic or diastolic wave is the reflection of impulse from the lower part of the body. With aging, hypertension and atherosclerosis there is reduced compliance of arterial tree, the tidal wave is accentuated and the diastolic wave is reduced (Fig. 1).

a. Hyperkinetic pulse (Large or Bounding pulse)
Hyperkinetic pulse indicates the rapid ejection of an increased volume of blood from the left ventricle (LV). This is more prominent in brachial, radial and femoral arteries than in the carotid artery (Table 2).

Water hammer pulse: It refers to an extremely rapid forceful ascending limb of the arterial pulse wave.

Collapsing pulse: It refers to quick marked decrease in the arterial pulse wave following its peak (descending limb).

Quincke pulse: Small visible pulsations in the nail bed of patients with hyper dynamic arterial pulse of any cause.

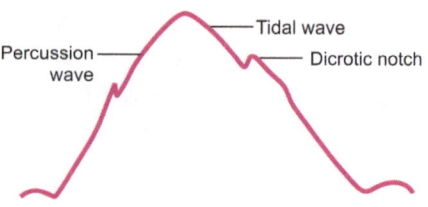

Figure 1 Normal arterial pulse

Table 2
Causes of hyperkinetic pulse

HYPERKINETIC PULSE
Aortic regurgitation
Persistent ductus arteriosus
Arteriovenous fistula Ruptured sinus of valsalva
Persistent truncus arteriosus
Large aorta and collaterals in pulmonary atresia
Thyrotoxicosis
Severe cirrhosis
Anemia
Pregnancy

Usually in hyperkinetic pulse, the pulse pressure is wide. Rapid rate of rise of the pulse without a wide pulse pressure is called brisk pulse, or small collapsing pulse seen in mitral regurgitation (MR) and ventricular septal defect (VSD).

Hyperkinetic pulse is seen in normal people during hyperkinetic circulatory states like fever, exercise and with marked bradycardia associated with increased stroke volume as in Athletes. Abnormal rapid run off of blood from the arterial system also produce hyperkinetic pulse (Fig. 2).

Pulse in Aortic Regurgitation

The pulse wave in aortic regurgitation is called as *Collapsing pulse,* which refers to a rapid decent of the pulse wave. This is because there is **a rapid decrease in the rate of ejection during systole, that is seen in patients with aortic regurgitation**. In addition, there is a **rapid emptying of the arterial system due to marked increase in the velocity of the bloodstream.** Blood leaking back into the LV in aortic regurgitation is a diastolic phenomena and not a systolic one.

b. Hypokinetic Pulse
This is a small amplitude pulse resulting from decreased LV stroke volume with decreased LV ejection time, as there is less

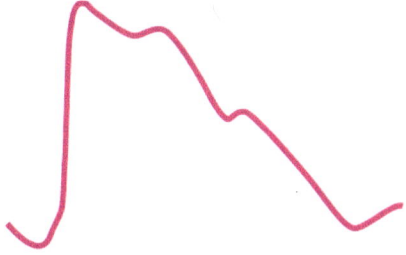

Figure 2 Hyperkinetic pulse: Abrupt upstroke (percussion wave) followed by rapid collapse later in systole

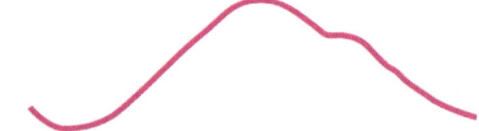

Figure 3 Hypokinetic pulse: Small amplitude with slow upstroke

blood to eject. Causes include LV dysfunction, overt congestive cardiac failure, hypotensive states like hypovolemia, left ventricular outflow tract (LVOT) obstruction. The rate of rise of the hypokinetic pulse is important. If it is prolonged it suggests LVOT obstruction (Fig. 3).

Pulsus Parvus et Tardus

It is a small amplitude pulse with delayed systolic peak. Occasionally, there may be a detectable shoulder on the upstroke of the carotid pulse, (the anacrotic shoulder). Palpable coarse vibrations present as systolic thrill is often felt over the slowly rising carotid pulse (Fig. 4).

Anacrotic pulse refers to an exaggerated anacrotic notch found in aortic stenosis—the notch may be related to a jet effect produced by ejection across the abnormal valve or to decreased velocity of flow during ejection. This is not usually palpable but is recordable.

C. Bisferiens Pulse

This is twice beating pulse with **two positive waves in systole**. Abnormalities of LV ejection and reflected waves from the periphery contribute to the prominence of tidal wave. It is associated with ejection of a rapid jet of blood through the aortic valve (Table 3).

Mechanism: (Peter Fleming; BMJ 19; 519). At the peak of flow, Bernoulli effect (suction effect of a rapid flow over a surface) on the walls of ascending aorta causes a sudden decrease in the arterial pressure on the inner aspect of the wall.

It is **best felt in the carotid**; sometimes more easily felt in the brachial or radial artery.

This condition is more likely to be present with larger stroke volume and hence may disappear with the onset of ventricular dysfunction in aortic regurgitation (Fig. 5).

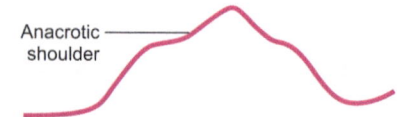

Figure 4 Pulsus parvus et tardus: Small pulse with delayed systolic peak

Table 3
Causes of bisferiens pulse

BISFERIENS PULSE
Severe aortic regurgitation
Moderate aortic stenosis with severe aortic regurgitation
Hypertrophic cardiomyopathy
Patent ductus arteriosus
Exercise
Fever
Rarely in normal individuals

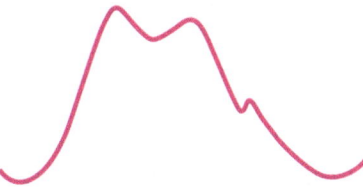

Figure 5 Bisferiens pulse: Two systolic peak, the percussion and tidal waves separated by a distinct mid systolic dip; the peak may be equal, or either may be larger

In hypertrophic cardiomyopathy, bisferiens pulse is often recorded but not palpated and most of them have a pressure gradient in the LVOT. The mid systolic negative wave coincides with the marked reduction in the rate of LV ejection. The height of percussion wave is greater than that of the tidal wave in most instances. On palpation often there is a rapid upstroke, or the arterial pulse is normal or simple hyperkinetic, but inhaling amyl nitrite or performing valsalva manoeuvre can elicit obstruction and bisferiens. A finding nearly specific for hypertrophic cardiomyopathy is a much smaller arterial pressure pulse in the cycle following a ventricular premature beat. This pulse is also called **bifid** or **spike** and **dome pulse** (Fig. 6).

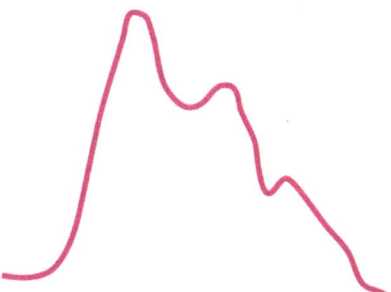

Figure 6 Spike and dome pulse

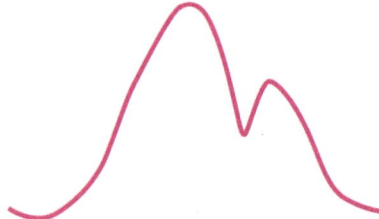

Figure 7 Dicrotic pulse: Two peaks but second peak is in diastole not to be confused with bisferiens pulse, in which both the peaks occur in systole

d. Dicrotic Pulse

The dicrotic (from Greek, **dickrotos** means double beating) pulse is a twice-peaked pulse with one peak in systole and second peak in diastole, the latter, due to an accentuated and palpable dicrotic wave that follows the second heart sound. It is best felt in carotids; it may also be palpated over more peripheral arteries (Fig. 7). Abnormalities are (i) short ejection phase, (ii) low dicrotic notch, (iii) a large diastolic wave, (iv) a narrow pulse pressure, (v) a diminished rate of rise of pulse, and (vi) lack of distinct percussion and tidal waves. In general it is not observed over 45 years (as arterial tree is inelastic) (Table 4).

Table 4
Causes of dicrotic pulse

Cardiomyopathy or severe LV dysfunction
Following valve replacement for AR or MR (indicates poor LV function)
Febrile states in young subjects (controversial)
During inspiration in pericardial tamponade

Pulsus Alternans

These are beats that occur at regular intervals with regular alternation of the systolic height of the pressure pulses. Rarely the weaker pulse is not felt at all (total alternans). Sustained pulsus alternans is due to alteration of the contractile state of at least part of the myocardium, which may be caused by the failure of electromechanical coupling in some cells during the weaker contraction. The subsequent stronger contraction would then mean contraction of all cells, some of which were potentiated. It is better appreciated by **palpating a distal artery** with a slightly wider pulse pressure than the carotid artery and is often brought out or accentuated in upright position or taking nitroglycerine tablet due to decreased venous return. Respiration should be held during the examination. It can be confirmed using sphygmomanometer (Fig. 8).

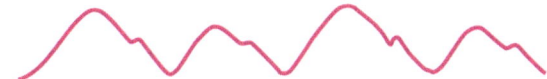

Figure 8 Pulsus alternans: Alternate strong and weak pulse and characterized by regular rhythm and must be distinguished from pulses bigeminus which is usually irregular

Causes

LV failure produced by severe hypertension, aortic valve disease, coronary atherosclerosis or cardiomyopathy. *Concordant pulsus alternans*—pulmonary artery pulsus alternans occurring simultaneously with the aortic pulsus alternans.

Different types of pulses alternans
1. Pulsus alternans: Regular alternation of strong and weak pulses in the absence of respiratory or cycle length alteration.
2. Total alternans: When the weak contraction fails to open the aortic valve, alternate pulses may be absent.
3. Independent alternans: Pure alternans of Right or left ventricle.
4. Concordant alternans: Right—left ventricle alternate together.
5. Discordant alternans: Right—left ventricles alternate alternatingly.
6. Compound alternans: Further alternation of the weaker beats occurs superimposed on the routine alternans.

Pulsus Bigeminus

These are alternating strong and weak pulses, occurring with an irregular rhythm, seen in supraventricular or ventricular bigemini.

Pulsus Paradoxus

It is defined as a marked decrease in pulse amplitude during normal quiet inspiration or a decrease in the systolic arterial pressure by more than 10 mm Hg (Table 5).

Table 5
Causes of pulsus paradoxus

Cardiac tamponade
Emphysema
Asthma
Marked obesity
Severe congestive cardiac failure
Constrictive pericarditis

It may be produced by conditions which are as follows:
1. Limit the inspiratory increase in blood flow to the RV and pulmonary artery.
2. Cause greater than normal pooling of blood in the lungs during inspiration.
3. Cause the intrathoracic pressure to have very wide fluctuations during inspiration and expiration.
4. Interfere with venous return to either atrium relatively more during inspiration.

The term pulsus paradoxus is a misnomer because systolic BP falls slightly during inspiration normally. To elicit pulsus paradoxus, comfortably position the patient. Ask the patients to breathe as regularly and quietly as comfort permits. Apply thumb to the brachial pulse with enough pressure to elicit maximum systolic impact. Release the pressure till the pulse disappears on inspiration. Sphygmomanometer cuff is deflated at 2–3 mm Hg per heartbeat. Identify the peak systolic pressure during expiration. Deflate the cuff very slowly in order to precisely identify the pressure at which korotkoff sounds become audible during inspiration and expiration. When difference is more than 10 mm Hg during quiet respiration, pulsus paradoxus is present.

In cardiac tamponade, increased intrapericardial pressure leads to decreased filling capacity of heart. During inspiration, expected augmentation of venous return to the right side occurs. Decreased thoracic pressure causes pooling of blood in pulmonary veins and capillaries and decreases the venous return to left atrium. The increased right sided volume leads to an obligatory decrease in left side heart filling as the total cardiac filling capacity is limited. This leads to decreased stroke volume and decreased systolic BP in inspiration. In emphysema, bronchial asthma and pulmonary embolism, wide swings of intrathoracic pressure is the mechanism. Marked obesity causes increased work of breathing which may explain the pulsus paradoxus. In severe CCF, tension on the heart and pericardium produced by downward movement of diaphragm during inspiration pulls the heart inferiorly leading to increased intra pericardial pressure. Superior vena caval obstruction and constrictive pericarditis are rare causes.

Reverse pulsus paradoxus may be seen in intermittent positive pressure ventilation (IPPV) and isorythmic AV dissociation.

Causes of Reversed Pulsus paradoxus
- **IPPV:** Intrathoracic pressure is higher in inspiration and lower in expiration
- **Isorhythmic AV dissociation:** The atrial activity precedes the ventricular activity during inspiration and follows it during expiration
- **HCM**—exact mechanism not known.

VOLUME OF PULSE

The amplitude of excursion of the pulse is used to assess the volume of pulse and generally correlates with stroke volume. In elderly with rigid atherosclerotic aorta and in systemic hypertension the pulse volume is high due to nondistensible arterial system. In these settings, the pulse volume is not a true reflector of stroke volume (Tables 6 and 7).

RADIOFEMORAL DELAY

In a normal adult, the pulse transmission from aorta to carotid, femoral, brachial and radial artery occurs at 30 msec, 75 msec, 65 msec, 80 msec, respectively. When coarctation of aorta is suspected it desirable to examine the radial and femoral pulse simultaneously to assess radiofemoral delay. Some prefer brachio-femoral delay as there is an already existing delay between brachial and femoral and with further delay it is easily made out.

Method of Examination

- Make the patient lie down supine
- Place the patients right arm straight, parallel and close to the body
- Place the left hand of the examiner at the radial artery
- Place the right index finger of the examiner at the right femoral artery of the patient.

The idea is that you must examine the femoral artery and the radial artery as close as possible, in one line. If you keep the patients hand faraway from the patients femoral artery then you will not appreciate the delay better.

Table 6
Causes of high-volume pulse

Hyperkinetic heart syndrome
High cardiac output states, e.g. anemia, thyrotoxicosis
Emotional excitability and anxiety
Conditions with aortic run off
Systemic hypertension
Elderly

Table 7
Causes of low-volume pulse

Shock
Low cardiac output
a. Myocardial disease
b. Valvular disease
c. Pericardial disease
Acute hypertension as in eclampsia of pregnancy

In coarctation of aorta the peak of the femoral artery pulse is delayed. This is something similar to the aortic stenosis, in which there is a delayed peak. In fact we are actually comparing the delayed peak of the femoral pulse with the radial pulse. Kindly note that it is not a delayed arrival, but delayed peak.

CONDITION OF VESSEL WALL

While examining the peripheral arterial pulse, it is desirable to assess the rigidity and elasticity of the arteries. The rigidity of the arterial pulse is best appreciated by examining the femoral, radial, brachial and carotid pulses. In clinical practice the thickness and firmness of the arterial wall are examined by rolling the vessel, usually the radial artery, against the underlying tissue. The more rigid the artery, the less it is compressible. In order to appreciate nonelastic, rigid peripheral arteries it is desirable to perform **Osler's maneuver**.

This is done by elevating the cuff pressure to obliterate the radial pulse and, if upon obliteration of the pulse, the radial artery easily palpable and appears rigid (positive Osler's sign) then there might be a significant difference between indirect measurement of arterial pressure by cuff method and directly determined intra arterial pressure.

Three-finger method: The index, middle and fourth finger of the left hand are used for palpating the radial pulse. With the index finger occlude the ulnar collateral, by compressing the artery distally. Compress the radial artery with the fourth finger thus occluding the flow into the artery. Now, use the middle finger to roll the artery and palpate its thickness.

The only condition that pathologically makes the radial artery thick is Monkeberg's sclerosis.

CHAPTER 3

Blood Pressure

Oomen K George

CHAPTER OUTLINE

- Methods of Measuring Arterial Blood Pressure
- Korotkoff Sounds (KS)
- AHA Recommendations
- Features Indicative of Secondary Causes
- Guidelines for Measuring BP
- Valsalva Maneuver and Blood Pressure
- Ambulatory BP Monitoring – ABPM
- BP Thresholds – Definition 28
- Goals in Hypertenson – JNC 2014

The arterial blood pressure is a measure of the *lateral force per unit area* of vascular wall. It is quantified as mm of Hg or dynes/cm.

White Coat Hypertension

Blood pressure is more than 140/90 when measured in office, but less than 135/85 during day time ambulatory recording. The usual prevalence is 15–30% of the population. This is more common in the elderly.

Pseudohypertension

With increasing age, the vessel wall gets thickened and the blood pressure cuff does not obliterate the arterial wall properly and there can be higher blood pressure recordings. This is called as pseudohypertension.

Orthostatic Hypotension

BP is measured in supine position, immediately after standing and within 3 minutes after standing. *A 20 mm drop in systolic BP or 10 mm drop in diastolic BP is defined as orthostatic hypotension.*

METHODS OF MEASURING ARTERIAL BLOOD PRESSURE

A. Direct Method

In this, a catheter is passed into the artery and the pressure is measured directly.

B. Indirect Method

Invention of the pneumatic cuff manometer (Riva, Rocci-1896) and Korotkoff sounds (1905) permitted indirect measurement of arterial blood pressure.

KOROTKOFF SOUNDS (KS)

This represents oscillations of the partially occluded arterial wall as a result of distension with each cardiac impulse.

Five Phases

1. Phase I: Clear tapping sounds occur when cuff pressure has fallen to arterial peak systolic level.
2. Phase II: Murmurs of swishing sounds occurs at least 10–15 mm Hg below peak systolic pressure.
   Auscultatory gap is the period of abnormal silence or diminished intensity of Phase IIKS. The pulse is palpable during this time. This is seen in 5% of people. The Korotkoff sounds reappear at a pressure 10–20 mm Hg lower than the systolic blood pressure.
3. Phase III: Loud.
4. Phase IV: Muffling.
5. Phase V: Complete cessation of sounds.

AHA RECOMMENDATIONS (TABLE 1)

Systolic BP is recorded at the point where tapping **sounds are heard** for two consecutive beats and DBP is at the point where Korotkoff sounds is **inaudible.**

In patients with aortic regurgitation, phase IV is to be taken as the DBP.

It is recommended that the width of the bladder be 40% at arm circumference, and the length of the bladder be long enough to encircle at least 80% of the arm in adults. In

Table 1
AHA recommendations for BP cuff dimensions

	Mid-arm circumference (cm)	Bladder width (cm)	Bladder length (cm)
Newborn	5–7.5	3	5
Infant	7.5–13	5	8
Child	13–20	8	13
Small adult	17–26	11	17
Adult	24–32	13	24
Large adult	34–42	17	32
Thigh	42–50	20	42

children, the occluding bladder should be long enough to encircle the arm completely (100%). Overlapping the ends of the bladder in children doesn't appear to introduce an error in measurement.

The British Hypertension Society has recommended the use of one large cuff, width 12.5–13 cm and length 35 cm, for all adults with an arm circumference, exceeding 33 cm in order to avoid the need for multiple cuff sizes.

FEATURES INDICATIVE OF SECONDARY CAUSES

1. Onset of hypertension before the age of 20 or after 50 years of age.
2. Blood pressure of >180/110.
3. Abdominal bruit.
4. Unexplained hypokalemia.
5. Varying blood pressures with sweating, tremor.

GUIDELINES FOR MEASURING BP

Posture

1. Usually blood pressure is recorded in a resting stage. Preferable to do the same after 3 minutes of rest in a **sitting** posture.
2. **Arm position:** The recommended position is patients' elbow at the level of the heart usually 4th intercostal space at the sternum. If the patients arm is higher by 6 cm, the systolic and diastolic pressure will be around 5mm Hg lower. These errors are explained by hydrostatic effect.
   It is essential that the arm is supported during blood pressure measurement. This is best achieved in practice by having the observer hold the arm at the elbow.
3. Which arm? For the first time, you should measure in both the arms. If the difference is more than 20 mm of Hg for systolic and 10 for diastolic between both the arms then the patient needs further evaluation. It has been our preference to use the **right arm**.

Circumstances

1. No caffeine for preceding hour.
2. No smoking for preceding 15 minutes.
3. No exogenous adrenergic stimulants, e.g., phenylephrine in nasal decongestants or eye drops for pupillary dilation.
4. A quite, warm setting.
5. Home readings taken under varying circumstances and 24-hour ambulatory recordings may be preferable and more accurate in predicting subsequent cardiovascular disease.

Equipment

1. *Cuff size:* You must use appropriate cuff size. Refer the Table 1 for AHA recommendations for BP cutt dimensions.
2. **Manometer**: Aneroid gauges should be calibrated every 6 months against a mercury manometer. The manometer should not be more than 3 feet (92 cms) so that the scale can be read easily. The mercury column should be vertical and at eye level.
3. **For infants**: Use ultrasound equipment, e.g., the Doppler method.

Technique

1. On each occasion, take at least two readings, separated by as much time as is practical. If readings vary by more than 5 mm Hg, take additional readings until two are close.
2. For diagnosis, obtain at least 3 sets of readings at least a week apart.
3. Inflate the bladder quickly to a pressure 20 mm Hg above the systolic, as recognized by disappearance of the radial pulse and deflate the bladder 3 mm Hg every second.

VALSALVA MANEUVER AND BLOOD PRESSURE

Force expiration against a closed glottis for 20 seconds.

Technique
- Ask the patient to blow into the tubing of the BP machine to a pressure of 40 mm of Hg for 30 seconds
- Apply firm pressure over the abdomen and ask him to resist your inward pressure.

The normal response consists of four phases (Fig. 1).
1. *Phase* I: Systolic and diastolic pressures will rise proportionate to rise in intrathoracic pressure.
2. *Phase* II: Systolic and diastolic pressures will fall because of reduced venous return.
3. *Phase* III: Immediately after release, there is an abrupt transient decrease in arterial pressure.
4. *Phase IV:* There is an overshoot of pressures and reflex bradycardia (Table 2).

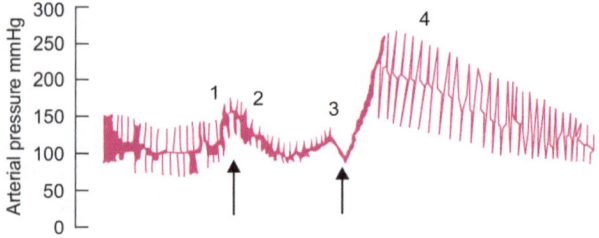

Figure1 Different phases of Valsalva maneuver

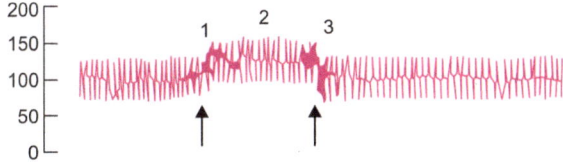

Figure 2 Square-wave response of BP in CCF during Valsalva maneuver

Table 2
ESC 2013 classification

Category	SBP	DBP
Normal	120–129 and	80–84
High Normal	130–139	85–89
Grade 1	140–159	90–99
Grade 2	160–179	100–109
Grade 3	>180	>110
Isolated Systolic	>140 and	<90

In CCF there is square wave response of BP to Valsalva maneuver. Throughout the strain phase BP stays up and there is no overshoot response on release of the valsalva (Fig. 2).

AMBULATORY BP MONITORING (ABPM)

Indications for ABPM

- White coat HTN, masked HTN or paroxysmal HTN
- Increased BP variability
- Resistant HTN
- OSA
- Low BP/Orthostatic hypotension
- To assess the efficacy of antihypertensive drugs.

BP THRESHOLDS—DEFINITION

Given in Table 3 is the various cutoff values that are used in the definition.
- Definition of dipping: during 24 ABPM : Night time BP/Daytime BP ratio: No Dipping: If > 1.will have more risk of CV events; Excessive dipping: if < 0.8. will have more risk of stroke.

GOALS IN HYPERTENSON—JNC 2014[1]

- Age more than 60: BP goal is lower than 150/90
- Age less than 60: BP goal is lower than 140/90
- All ages diabetes with or without CKD lower than140/90
- All ages CKD with or without DM lower than 140/90.

Table 3
Hypertension thresholds (ESC 2013)

	Systolic	Diastolic
Clinic	140	90
24 hour	130	80
Day	135	85
Night	120	70
Home	135	85

REFERENCE

1. Paul AJ et al. Evidence based guideline for the management of high blood pressure. JAMA. Feb 2014.

CHAPTER 4

Jugular Venous Pulse

Oomen K George, Bobby John

CHAPTER OUTLINE

- Definition
- Abnormalities of X Descent
- Determination of Jugular venous Pulse
- Abnormalities of Y Descent
- Technique of Examination
- Atrial Septal Defect
- Difference between Venous and Arterial Pulsation
- Tricuspid Regurgitation
- Normal Wave Pattern
- Constrictive Pericarditis
- Hepatojugular Reflux
- Eisenmenger Syndrome
- Abnormalities of a Wave
- Cyanotic Heart Disease

Potain first described jugular venous waveforms, but it was James Mackenzie who named the waves and firmly established the Jugular venous pulse (JVP) as an important part of clinical examination.

DEFINITION

Jugular venous pulse is defined as the oscillating top of the column of blood in the proximal portion of the internal jugular vein and represents volumetric changes that faithfully reflects the right atrial pressures at all stages of cardiac cycle.

DETERMINATION OF JVP

A. *Internal jugular vein (IJV) is preferred to External jugular vein (EJV) for measurement of JVP for the following reasons:*
1. IJV is in direct line with superior vena cava (SVC) and right atrium (RA).
2. External Jugular vein possesses valves that may interfere with the measurement of venous pressure. Internal jugular vein also has a valve just above its junction with the subclavian vein; however, it is only a functional valve, which acts when intrathoracic pressure is elevated suddenly as in coughing.
3. EJV passes through multiple fascial planes unlike IJV.
4. EJV is often not visible due to vasoconstriction especially in shock like states.

5. The external jugular vein is not pulsatile as a rule but instead often presents as a visible column that distends to a crest, which is a reliable measure of mean right atrial pressure.

B. *The right IJV is preferred to the left IJV for the following reasons:*

1. The direct communication of the right internal jugular vein through the right innominate vein and superior vena cava is in a straight-line renders it better susceptible to the pressure changes of the right heart.
2. Partial obstruction of the left innominate vein from compression between the aortic arch and the sternum particularly in elderly impairs transmission of right atrial pressures to the left internal jugular vein.
3. The presence of a left SVC draining into coronary sinus will cause a slightly higher pressure in the left than right possibly due to greater emptying resistance. This is especially important in ASD.

The Jugular venous pulse should be clinically analyzed in terms of pressure and waveforms. The central venous pressure is influenced by the volume of blood in the venous system, venous tone, right atrial contraction and relaxation, closure of the tricuspid valve, right ventricular diastolic tone and intrathoracic pressure.

TECHNIQUE OF EXAMINATION

- Patient should be lying comfortably preferably in a bed or examination table that permits controlled elevation of trunk above the horizontal.
- The higher the central venous pressure, the higher the elevation required from the horizontal. Start with 30-degree elevation above horizontal and adjust position till the upper end of venous pulsations become visible. The patients with low venous pressures have waveforms visible only in or just below horizontal. The patient's head is adjusted and turned slightly, not tensing the sternomastoid.
- A small light should be shone tangentially across the area so that the shadows of the EJV and IJV are cast. Left hand is used to adjust the light source leaving the right hand to palpate the left carotid artery or for applying the stethoscope.

Methods to Make JVP More Obvious

1. Inspiration often makes the JVP more obvious. This is chiefly so because the descents, especially the "x" descent becomes brisker and more apparent to the eye. Intrathoracic pressure falls during inspiration and mean atrial and jugular venous pressures decline hence during inspiration JVP is more readily seen but at a lower mean level.

2. Horizontal posture—more effective if the legs are raised.
3. Leg binders.
4. Overalls that can be inflated.
5. IV infusions.

DIFFERENCES BETWEEN THE VENOUS AND ARTERIAL PULSATIONS

Table 1 differentiates between venous and arterial pulsations.

Table 1
Differences in venous and arterial pulsations

S. No.	Venous pulsation	Arterial pulsation
1	Movement is soft, diffuse and undulant	Movement is pulsatile
2	Better seen than felt	Better felt
3	There are two crests and two troughs	There is only one upstroke and descent
4	The descent (x) is rapid	The descent is slow
5	Fastest movement is collapse or descent	Fastest movement is the upstroke
6	Firm pressure just above the clavicle obliterates	Firm pressure just above the clavicle does not obliterate.
7	Varies with inspiration, posture or abdominal compression	Does not vary with inspiration, posture or abdominal compression
8	This is situated laterally	This is situated medially

NORMAL WAVE PATTERN (FIG. 1)

The JVP consists of essentially four waves—*a*, *x*, *v* and *y*. The *a* wave and *v* wave are crests, the *x* wave and *y* wave are troughs. A fifth wave known as *c* wave, another crest, may interrupt *x* descent. A plateau before *c* wave is called *z* point.

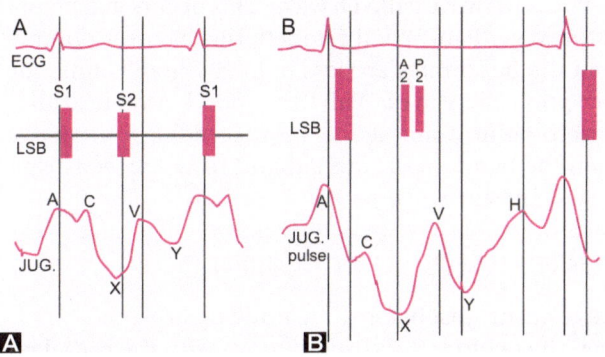

Figure 1 (A) Normal jugular pulse tracings, showing the various wave forms; (B) The h wave is seen; this wave is well seen in slow heart rate

a Wave

The *a* wave is due to the **atrial systole**. It is the dominant wave occurring before the carotid arterial pulse and first heart sound.

x Descent

The *x* descent is initiated by **the atrial relaxation**. The rest of the descent after *c* wave, is due to the **descent of atrial floor** as the tricuspid annulus is pulled caudally by the ventricular contraction. *x* descent starts during systole and ends just before S2.

c Wave

The *c* wave occurs in the x descent and is due to the **carotid artefact** and pushing up of the tricuspid valve with ventricular contraction.

v Wave

The ascending limb of the *v* wave reflects passive **filling of the right atrium** in the face of closed tricuspid valve (during ventricular systolic). It begins late in systole and ends in early diastole. This roughly synchronous with the carotid pulse, and peaks just after S2

y Descent

The *y* descent is due to sudden termination of *v* wave as right ventricle relaxes and tricuspid valve opens at the end of the period of isometric ventricular relaxation. The *y* descent begins and ends during diastole.

h Wave

Following *y* trough, the filling of both right atrial and ventricles occurs and pressure rises gradually to form a small brief positive wave called *h* wave. This occurs just before the next *a* wave. Paul Wood refers to this as the *z* point. Only when the heart rates are less than 90, there is time for the inscription all 5 waves. With heart rates between 90 and 110, the zero point is not defined, a succeeding y immediately. When the heart rate is more than 110, *a* succeeds *y* just as the descent starts.

TEMPORAL SEQUENCE WITH CARDIAC CYCLE

a wave occurs just before S1/carotid upstroke
x wave just **before S2 (simultaneous with the radial pulse)**
v wave after carotid upstroke
y wave after S2.

NORMAL JUGULAR VENOUS PRESSURE

With the patient's trunk elevated to 40° above the horizontal, the crest of normal a and v waves do not exceed 3–4 cm above the angle of Louis. At 45° the upper limit of the normal venous pressure is 4.5 cm above the sternal angle. The addition of 5 cm to the level of the venous pressure at the sternal angle obtains a right catheter equivalent pressure, in centimetres of water.

ELEVATED JUGULAR VENOUS PRESSURE

The best definition of elevated JVP is that of Sir Thomas Lewis. He defines it as an elevation of the top of the external or internal jugular veins more than 3 cm of vertical distance above the sternal angle of Louis.

Phlebostatic axis of Burch: A line representing the intersection of the cross sectional plane through the fourth intercostal space at the sternum and the coronal plane midway between the back and xiphoid is called the *Phlebostatic axis of Burch*. This line traverses the posterior right atrium in most individuals.

Significance: The venous pressure of healthy adults changes less than 1–2 cm water whether the individual is supine, prone or in various positions between supine and upright.

CAUSES OF ELEVATED JVP

1. CCF.
2. Increased blood volume.
3. Increased intrathoracic, intrapericardial or intra-abdominal pressures.
4. Tricuspid stenosis.
5. Partial obstruction of SVC.
6. Hyperkinetic circulatory states.
7. Space occupying lesions affecting the right side of the heart.
8. Slow heart rate.
9. Excitement.
10. Effort.

HEPATOJUGULAR REFLUX (PASTEUR RONDOT MANEUVER)

- This was described in 1885 first by Pasteur in tricuspid regurgitation (Pasteur W. Note on a new physical sign of tricuspid regurgitation. Lancet. 1885;2:524)
- Rondot described it in CCF. Abdominal compression initially results in an increased venous return while continued pressure is accompanied by a fall in the IVC flow and rise in femoral venous pressure. (**Note the term**

reflux than reflex since no neurons are involved. BMJ. May 1999)

Technique

- The palm of the right hand with fingers apart is applied over the center of the abdomen
- Duration of pressure: **15 seconds**
- Amount of pressure: 20–35 mm of Hg.

Normal Response

There is a transient increase of JVP for a few beats (for 10 sec) followed by fall to a control level as the abdominal pressure continues. In the presence of RV failure, the initial rise in JVP is not followed promptly by a fall but instead is maintained during the entire period of compression. **A rise of at least 3 cm for 15 seconds is a positive hepatojugular reflux** (Am J Medicine. 2000;109:59).

HJR is Positive in

1. Constriction
2. Restriction
3. RV MI
4. LV failure if Wedge is more than 15 mm Hg.

False-positive Hepatojugular Reflux

1. Severe COPD (due to disproportionate increase in intra thoracic pressures)
2. Increased blood volume

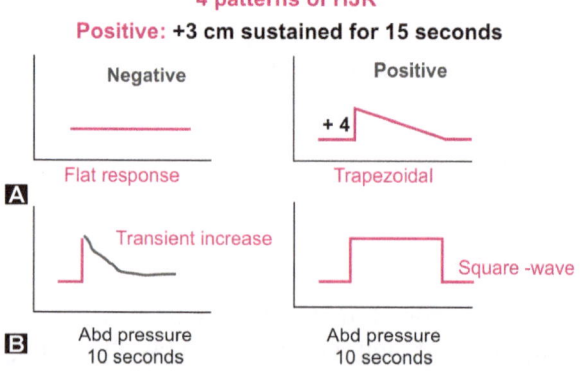

Figure 2 Response of abdominal pressure can be positive or negative. Negative responses are shown on left and positive responses are shown in right (*Adapted from* (A) American Journal of Medicine 2000;109:59; (B) Annals of Internal Medicine 1998;109;456-60)

ALTERATION OF "a" WAVE

1. Giant *a* wave (Fig. 3 and Table 2))
Giant *a* waves occur when the right atrium contracts against an appreciable resistance at 2 levels – Tricuspid orifice, within cavity of RV, pulmonary stenosis, pulmonary regurgitation. Giant *a* waves are presystolic, abrupt, collapsing in quality, palpable, transmitted to the liver and usually associated with right atrial gallop and conspicuous p pulmonale. It measures 6–15 cm higher than the v waves—referred to as venous Corrigans.

2. Cannon waves (Fig. 4 and Table 3)
This occurs when the right atrium contracts against a closed tricuspid valve.

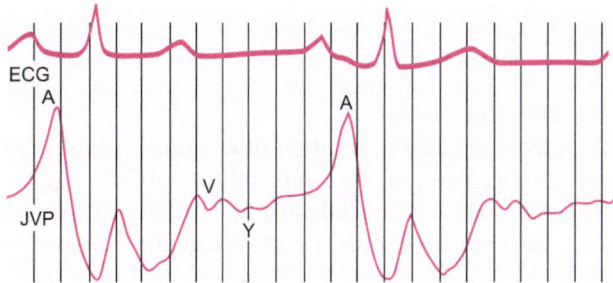

Figure 3 Jugular venous pulse in a patient with tricuspid stenosis in sinus rhythm showing large "a" wave, poorly-delineated v wave

Table 2
Causes of giant a wave

Severe pulmonary hypertension
Severe pulmonary stenosis
Bernheim's syndrome
Tricuspid stenosis Tricuspid atresia

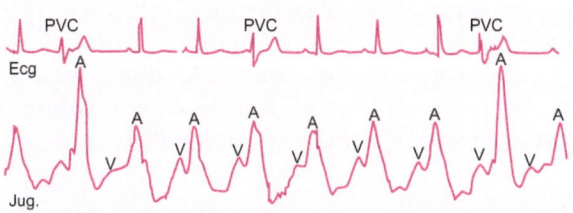

Figure 4 Jugular venous tracings showing cannon "a" waves due to premature ventricular complexes

Table 3
Causes of regular and irregular cannon 'a' waves

Regular	Irregular
Nodal rhythm	Complete heart block
Paroxysmal tachycardia	Multiple ectopic beats
Extremely prolonged PR interval	

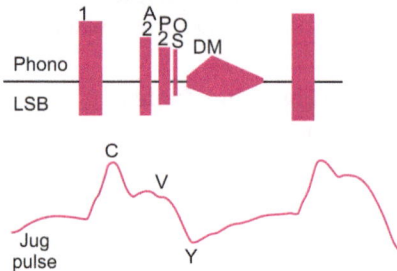

Figure 5 Jugular venous tracing showing absent a waves in a patient with mitral stenosis and atrial fibrillation

3. Absent a waves (Fig. 5)

The *a* waves are absent in atrial fibrillation whereas flutter waves can occasionally recognised in atrial flutter. *a* waves may also be absent when right atrium is dilated and does not possess effective mechanical systole, e.g. Ebstein's anomaly

Prolonged a-c Interval - Reflects PR interval.
It is graded into
    Short PR = 0.12 sec
    Average PR = 0.16 sec
    Long PR = 0.20 sec
    Obviously prolonged = 0.24 sec
When PR is more than 0.24 sec, *a* fuses with *v*.

X' DESCENT

x descent is typically lost in atrial fibrillation. It is blunted in tricuspid regurgitation.

Small x Descent

This condition is seen in when there is early build up of v wave with loss of capacitance of right atrium as when it is filled up by a tumor, loss of compliance of RA due to hypertrophy secondary to tricuspid stenosis, loss of pericardium that is seen in congenital absence or postoperative.

Prominent x Descent

The *x* descent is prominent with large *a* waves and increased right ventricular contraction as in pulmonary stenosis,

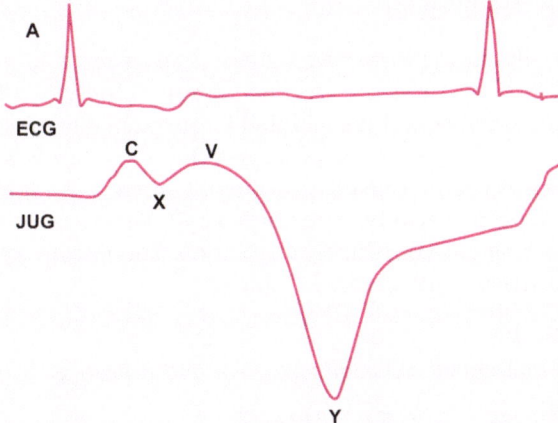

Figure 6 Jugular venous tracing showing prominent cv waves seen in patients with tricuspid insufficiency

pulmonary hypertension, ASD, Constrictive pericarditis, and cardiac tamponade.

v WAVE (FIG. 6)

Prominent v Waves

1. Typically in Tricuspid regurgitation (Lancisi's sign).
2. ASD due to excessive right atrial filling while tricuspid valve is closed.
3. Loss of compliance of right atrium as in constrictive pericarditis or after surgery.
4. Loss of pericardial attachment.
5. Hyperdynamic circulatory states.
6. Anomalous pulmonary venous drainage into right atrium.

y DESCENT

Slow y Descent

Typically in tricuspid stenosis, may also occur in the presence of severe RVH. The presence of steep y descent is a strong evidence against TS

Deep y Descent

Seen in constrictive pericarditis (Friedrich's Sign) TR and RV failure.

x versus y Descent

In PH, if the x is more than y descent – RV is compensated
If x is = y, then beginning of RV decompensation
If x is less than y then there is obvious RV decompensation.

KUSSMAUL'S SIGN

Normally during inspiration, there is an increase in *a* wave but a fall in venous pressure as a result of increased filling of right sided chambers with fall in intrathoracic pressures. An increase in JVP in inspiration when the heart is unable to accept the increased volume is known as Kussmaul's sign. This may also be contributed by the increase in intra-abdominal pressure during inspiration. This occurs typically in constrictive pericarditis (Table 4).

Table 4

Abnormal jugular wave form and clinical significance

Abnormal venous wave	*Clinical significance*
A wave	
Absent	Atrial fibrillation
Fused (with c wave)	Supraventricular tachycardia
Giant a wave	RA contraction against increased resistance 1. Tricuspid stenosis 2. Tricuspid atresia 3. Right atrial tumor Abnormal compliance of RV 1. Pulmonary stenosis 2. Pulmonary hypertension 3. Restrictive cardiomyopathy
Cannon wave	Isolated ventricular ectopics Regular – normal heart rate: Nodal rhythm Regular – rapid heart rate: Junctional tachycardia Irregular – Slow heart rate: Complete heart block Irregular – rapid heart rate: Ventricular tachycardia
x wave	
Absent	Tricuspid regurgitation
Large	Constrictive pericarditis, Restrictive cardiomyopathy, Atrial septal defect
v wave	
Large (fused with c wave)	Tricuspid regurgitation
y wave	
Slow descent	Tricuspid stenosis
Prominent rapid descent	Preceded by regurgitant systolic wave: Tricuspid regurgitation Not preceded by regurgitant systolic wave: Constrictive pericarditis (Friedreich's sign, restrictive cardiomyopathy, severe heart failure

Other causes
1. Right heart failure, e.g. RVMI.
2. RCMY.
3. Massive pulmonary embolism.
4. Partial obstruction of vena cavae.
5. Right atrial and right ventricular tumors.
6. TS.

SPECIFIC CARDIAC CONDITIONS

A. Atrial Septal Defect (Fig. 7)

In atrial septal defect *a* wave may be widened to as much as 0.18 sec. The *v* wave rises sharply and often taller than the *a* wave. There is a deep *x* due to contraction of dilated RV, tall *v* wave due to influx of left atrial blood and deep *y* descent due to discharge of large amount of blood into an enlarged compliant right ventricle.

B. Tricuspid Regurgitation

In tricuspid regurgitation, due to the disproportionate systolic filling of the right IJV which is in direct connection with the right atrium, right innominate vein and SVC results in right to left "head bob" best seen when the examiner observes the patient frontally.

C. Constrictive Pericarditis (Fig. 8)

1. In constrictive pericarditis, cardiac volume is set by the scarred pericardium and under no circumstances can the heart exceed this set volume, which is attained near the end of the first third of diastole.
2. During ejection, venous return is not significantly impeded; therefore the normal systolic surge of venous return, i.e. *v* wave and the *x* descent of venous pressure are preserved.

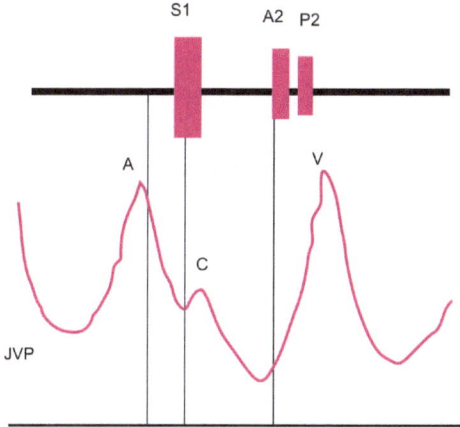

Figure 7 Schematic diagram of jugular venous pulse tracing in ASD showing prominent a and v wave with steep y descent

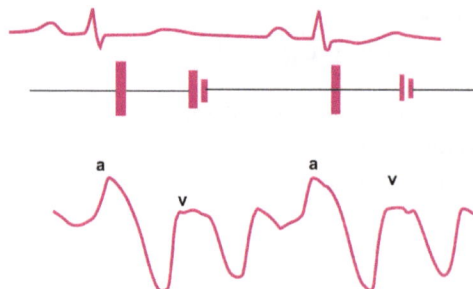

Figure 8 Jugular venous tracing showing deep x and y descents

3. Cardiac compression is still insignificant at end systole, so that when the tricuspid valve opens, blood rushes into the ventricle at a supernormal rate, registering a *y* descent of venous pressure.
4. Thus in constrictive pericarditis the venous filling is bimodal as in normal physiology, but the diastolic surge and *y* descent are equal or greater than the *x* descent, producing a 'W' pattern in JVP.

On the other hand, venous return in cardiac tamponade is unimodal and confined to ventricular systole which corresponds with the *x* descent of venous pressure. The *y* descent is therefore absent being replaced by an abnormal up sloping phase of the venous pressure pulse in early diastole.

D. Eisenmenger Syndrome

- Both venous pressure and pulse are commonly normal
- Small dominant "*a*" wave measuring 3 mm Hg is seen in 20–25% of cases of each type. A giant "*a*" wave measuring at least 6 mmHg is seen in 18% of cases with ASD, but rarely with VSD/PDA
- Large "*v*" wave from TR occurs in 5% of all cases.

E. Jugular Venous Wave Forms in Cyanotic Heart Disease (Table 5)

Table 5

Jugular waveforms in cyanotic heart disease

TOF or TOF like physiology	PS with Intact IVS with Right to Left shunt Atrial level	Tricuspid Atresia (TA)	Transposition with Increase PBF
Usually normal	• JVP Elevated • prominent "a" wave • v- normal • y descent prominent with associated TR	• JVP Elevated with restrictive ASD • Prominent "a" wave • "v" wave normal	• Elevated • "a" may be prominent • "v" normal

Precordial Examination— Palpation

Oomen K George

CHAPTER OUTLINE

- Apex Beat
- Point of Maximal Impulse (PMI)
- Character of Apical Impulse
- Sustained Apical Impulse
- Hyperdynamic Apical Impulse
- Hypokinetic Impulse
- Ectopic Impulse
- Parasternal Lift
- Epigastric Impulse
- Thrills
- Palpable Sounds

For optimal precordial examination, the room should be comfortably warm. The patient should be lying comfortably in the supine position or with the thorax elevated not more than 30 degrees.

Both the palm of the hand and the ventral surface of the proximal metacarpals and fingers should be used for palpation. The palm and the proximal metacarpals are preferred for initial localization of palpable cardiac motion and pads of fingers for precise localization and assessment of the impulse.

The pads of the fingers are most useful for detecting left ventricular (LV) and normal right ventricular (RV) motion. The palm and proximal metacarpals are usually best used for palpating larger, low frequency movements, such as the parasternal lift of right ventricular hypertrophy. Varying pressure with the hand is useful. High frequency movement such as ejection sounds, valve closure sounds, and mitral opening snaps are better detected with the hand held firmly against the chest, while low frequency movements such as ventricular diastolic filling events are best recognized with the finger tips. These subtle low-frequency motion of a palpable third heart sound (S3) or fourth heart sound (S4) or double systolic apical impulse will be felt only with light pressure of the fingers and may be missed, if palpated otherwise.

Before beginning systematic palpation, it is useful to observe the precordium for movements that are obvious at a glance. These movements can be enhanced by applying pen marks on the skin at the site under observation and by using a source of oblique illumination. The examiner should then look tangentially rather than from above. Parasternal movements are sometimes best seen when the examiner looks upward from the patient's feet. Precordial retraction is more readily seen than palpated, whereas outward displacement is more readily palpated than seen.

Timing of precordial events is best carried out using simultaneous palpation of the carotid arterial pulse with the left hand. Some find that concomitant auscultation of first heart sound (S1) and second heart sound (S2) is useful for timing purposes. Actual observation of the stethoscope head positioned directly on the apical impulse can help in identifying systole; S1 and early ejection occur synchronously with anterior motion of the stethoscope head.

In assessing the movements of the heart imparted to the chest wall, it is necessary to determine the *topographic location* of a given impulse as well as its *timing* in the cardiac cycle (early, mid or late systolic or diastole), its *duration* (how much of the cardiac cycle the impulse occupies), its displacement *characteristics* (vigor of movement, amplitude, and contour), and the maximum area occupied by the impulse (especially the LV impulse).

Palpation of the following 7 areas may be carried out systematically:

1. Apical Impulse—Point of maximal impulse.
2. Parasternal lift.
3. Epigastric area.
4. Pulmonary area.
5. Aortic area.
6. Sternoclavicular area.
7. Ectopic pulsations, if any.

APEX BEAT

Definition

The apex beat, otherwise called as cardiac impulse or apical thrust, is normally produced by left ventricular contraction. ***It is the lowermost and outermost point of definite cardiac impulse, which imparts a perpendicular thrust to the palpating finger.***

Mechanism

The palpable apical impulse in a normal subject is produced by an anterior movement of the LV during early systole. During the isovolumic contraction, ***the LV rotates in a counter clockwise direction along its long axis, and the*** *juxta-apical region lifts and makes contact with the anterior chest wall.*

Angiographic studies suggest that the interventricular septum (IVS) and the anteroseptal aspect of the LV make contact with the inner thoracic cage to form the palpable apical impulse. Following aortic valve opening, after the first half of ejection, the LV chamber moves away from the chest wall and the ventricle continues to decrease in size until systole is completed. Thus, the impulse felt on the precordium is comprised of an early, outward thrust, followed by retraction during the last part of systole. The retraction wave can be seen but is not felt.

Diastolic events, such as those produced by rapid LV filling (S3), or left atrial contraction (S4), are normally not palpable. With alterations in ventricular diastolic volume, pressure, or compliance, these events can be transmitted to the chest wall and may be felt by the examining fingers.

In the normal heart, the *apex* is on the left. The *inflow or sinus portion* of the RV underlies the fourth and fifth left intercostal spaces, while the *outflow portion* (infundibulum) underlies the third left interspace. The border of the *right atrium* (RA) is just lateral to the lower right sternal edge, and the *aortic root* (ascending aorta) is convex to the right of the sternum at the level of the second right interspace. The left atrium is not border forming because it is a posterior structure, except for its appendage, which underlies the third left interspace.

Characteristics of a normal apical impulse:
- A gentle nonsustained tap
- Early systolic anterior motion that ends before the last third of systole
- Located within 10 cm of the mid-sternal line in the 4th or 5th intercostals space
- A palpable area less than 2–2.5 sqcm and detectable in only one intercostals space
- RV motion is normally not palpable
- Diastolic events are normally not palpable
- May be completely absent in older persons.

Patient position: Palpation is best performed from the right side with upper trunk elevated at 30 degrees, both with the patient supine and in the partial left lateral decubitus position. Rotating to left lateral decubitus position with the left arm elevated over the head causes the heart to move laterally and increases the palpability of normal and pathological thrusts of the left ventricle.

The LV impulse is difficult to identify in the sitting position. In an occasional patient who would have to be examined in the sitting position, the impulse if palpable, can be relatively confidently related to the landmarks described above for the supine position.

Location: Normally the left ventricular impulse is medial and superior to the intersection of the left midclavicular line and the fifth intercostal space. In tall, thin persons, the apex beat can be distal (6th interspace) and more medial than usual. In infants and in adults with short, stocky chests, the impulse is often in the fourth left interspace.

It is within 10 cm of the midsternal line.

Displacement of the apex beat lateral to the midclavicular line *or more than 10cm lateral to the midsternal line* is a sensitive, but not specific *indicator of left ventricular enlargement*. The apical impulse may displaced upward and to the left by a high left diaphragm or during pregnancy. A tall, thin habitus has the opposite effect. Body build and thoracic configuration play a role in the displacement of the apical impulse. Scoliosis to the right rotates the heart leftward on its long axis; pectus excavatum shifts the heart to the left, altering the position of the normal left ventricular impulse. A decrease in anteroposterior chest dimensions (loss of thoracic kyphosis or shallow, saucer-shaped pectus excavatum) increases contact of the RV with the anterior chest wall.

Size: In the supine patient, the apex usually measures less than 2.5 cm and occupies only one interspace. In the left lateral decubitus position *diameter greater than 3 cm is an accurate sign of LV Enlargement.*

Duration: It is palpable as a single brief outward motion. It does not extend significantly into the left ventricular ejection phase. The outward movement of the apical impulse is felt only during first third of systole. Peak outward motion of the apical impulse occurs coincident with or just after aortic valve opening and the beginning of ejection. The beginning of the LV ejection at the bedside is appreciated by the onset of the carotid pulse upstroke. The impulse is sustained for a brief period (up to 0.08 sec) and then the outward movement ceases as the LV apex moves inward. The normal outward movement of the LV apical impulse recedes from the chest wall and becomes impalpable with the onset of ejection following the upstroke of the carotid pulse and during the downstroke of the carotid pulse. Thus, at the bedside when carotid pulse and left ventricular apical impulse are examined concurrently, these two impulse appear out of phase or asynchronous.

Amplitude: In normal individuals, the apex beat is a gentle outward motion. There may be respiratory alterations in the amplitude of the apex beat. Pay attention to the end of expiration if the impulse is hard to locate, although the peak amplitude may also occur during early inspiration.

Many older individuals do not commonly have palpable cardiac activity in the supine position. This may be due to an age related increase in the A–P thoracic diameter, an increase of muscle or fat on the chest wall. In most adults, LV activity can be detected when the subject is turned on to the left side, particularly in expiration. The causes of nonpalpable apical impulse are obesity, muscular chest wall, barrel chest, emphysema, coronary artery disease with decreased apical motion, pleural or pericardial effusion and age over 50 years.

Normal but hyperkinetic impulse: In anxious patients, there is often an increase in both the velocity and amplitude of the impulse, but not in its duration or area.

POINT OF MAXIMAL IMPULSE (PMI)

It need not necessarily be the apex beat, since the maximal precordial pulsation may be produced by an enlarged or hypertrophied RV, a dilated aorta or pulmonary artery, or a LV wall motion abnormality.

CHARACTER OF APICAL IMPULSE

The character of apical impulse is described in one of the following ones:
1. Normal.
2. Hyperkinetic.
3. Sustained.
4. Late systolic.
5. Hypokinetic.

SUSTAINED APICAL IMPULSE

The left ventricular heave or lift, which is more prominent in concentric hypertrophy, is characterized by a sustained outward movement of an area that is larger than the normal apex; i.e more than 2-3 cm in diameter and occupies more than one intercostal space. It is characterized by a prolonged **duration** of the outward movement extending into the ejection phase of the left ventricle. When the carotid pulse upstroke and duration are evaluated simultaneously with the left ventricular outward movement, the sustained apical impulse appears in phase with the carotid pulse upstroke and remains palpable during the down stroke of the carotid pulse. Often lasting upto the second heart sound, and this motion is accompanied by retraction of the left parasternal region. This rocking motion can often be appreciated by placing the index finger of one hand on the apex beat and that of the other hand in the parasternal region and by palpating the simultaneous out ward motion of the former while observing retraction of the latter (Fig. 1).

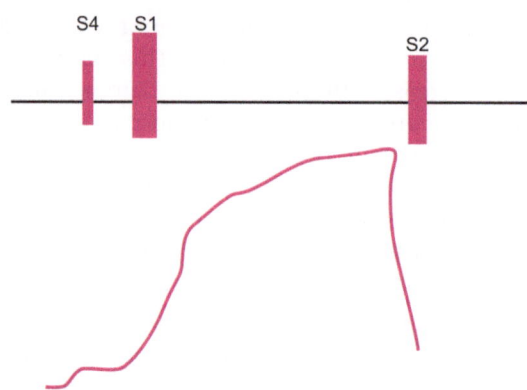

Figure 1 Schematic representation of sustained apical impulse

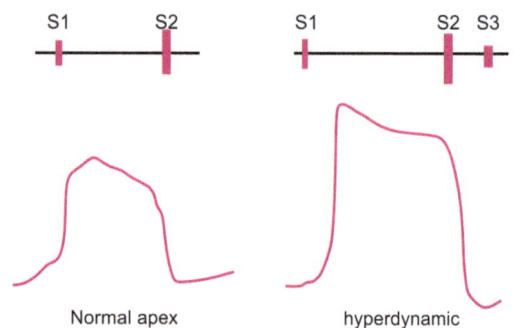

Figure 2 Schematic representation of normal and hyperdynamic apical cardiac impulse

HYPERDYNAMIC APICAL IMPULSE

There is increase in the **amplitude** of the LV impulse without a change in contour. The sequence between the onset of the carotid and the outward movement remains normal. It is appreciated as thrust of large amplitude that immediately disappears from the palpating fingers. When the duration of the ejection phase is estimated from the carotid pulse upstroke and down stroke or from the interval between first and second heart sound, the hyper dynamic apical impulse does not extend through out the systole (Fig. 2).

HYPOKINETIC IMPULSE

This is found in patient with reduced stroke volume, especially in acute myocardial infarction or dilated cardiomyopathy.

A sustained low amplitude impulse is called hypokinetic impulse. A hypokinetic LV impulse (low velocity and amplitude of systolic motion) is generally accompanied by reduced velocity and amplitude of medial retraction.

ECTOPIC IMPULSE

LV aneurysm may produce a sustained systolic bulge several centimeters superior to the left ventricular impulse, sometimes termed an *ectopic impulse*. It can be associated with a systolic impulse in unusual location, such as over the mid precordium. The most common site of an ectopic impulse is above and medial to the expected location of the LV impulse. The ectopic segment, often as readily seen as palpated, is usually caused by the anterior wall dyskinesia of coronary artery disease (CAD). LV aneurysm produces a larger than normal area of pulsation of the LV apex.

An anterolateral or apical aneurysm may be felt best at the apex but an anterior aneurysm may be felt several centimeters away from the apex. Some patients with dyskinetic left ventricles may have two distinct areas of rocking movement separated by several centimeters. Patients with LV aneurysm will have palpable 'a' wave, and thus a double apical impulse.

Anterior systolic movement of a normal RV can be caused by certain regional wall motion abnormalities of the LV. Dyskinetic motion of the ventricular septum during angina pectoris displaces the RV forward and results in a transient left parasternal impulse that disappears with relief of angina. In patient with angina pectoris, early systolic, late systolic or combined early and late systolic bulges can be occasionally appreciated at the bedside. If these abnormal apical impulses are transient and appreciated during anginal pain, reversible myocardial ischemia should be considered. This prolonged systolic impulse of regional dyskinesis is really "paradoxical" because it bulges abnormally during mid to late systole, at a time when normal, earlier anterior systolic movement has ceased.

Hypertrophic obstructive cardiomyopathy: A double systolic outward thrust of the left ventricle is characteristic of the patients with HOCM, who may also often exhibit a typical presystolic cardiac expansion, thus resulting in three separate outward movement of the chest wall during each cardiac cycle.

Constrictive pericarditis: When the left ventricle occupies the cardiac apex but the apex retracts in systole, the cause is usually chronic constrictive pericarditis. Retraction is usually most pronounced at the apex, but may extend as far as the left sternal edge. It is also characterized by systolic retraction of the ribs in the left axilla. (***Broadbent sign***). Prominent early diastolic left ventricular filling in constrictive pericarditis may be palpable. The precordial diastolic movement in chronic constrictive pericarditis has been called "diastolic heart beat". This is just as likely to be palpated over the RV as over the LV.

Diastolic motion: The outward motion of the apex characteristic of rapid LV diastolic filling is most readily palpated with the patient in the left lateral decubitus position and in full exhalation. This palpable equivalent of S3 is less often palpable than S4.

PARASTERNAL LIFT

Except in the first few months of life, right ventricle is not palpable. In children and in occasional adults with thin chest walls, a brief, gentle impulse may be palpable over the left third and fourth interspaces. This impulse is usually in diastole. Although the RV, located just beneath the sternum and left 3rd to 5th ribs, is closer to the chest wall than the left ventricle, RV activity is not normally felt. This is probably because the RV is thin walled (2-3 mm wall thickness), low pressure (20-25 mm Hg peak systolic pressure), and it pulls away from the anterior chest as the heart rotates in a counter clockwise fashion in early systole.

Parasternal lift: (Replacing systolic retraction) in the left parasternal region, best felt by the proximal palm or fingertips and with the patient supine, usually represents RV enlargement or hypertrophy.

1. The patient should rest supine at 30 degrees.
2. It is desirable to use **held end expiration** for RV examination. Movements of the examining hands and fingers should be carefully observed, as the typical low amplitude RV activity is better seen than felt. RV abnormalities are only detectable in the supine position.
3. Firm downward pressure with the hand on the lower left sternal area is usually necessary. Since RV activity is usually low amplitude, it will not be detected without such firm compression.

Two methods of RV palpation are recommended:
1. The **heel of the hand** can be applied firmly to the left sternal edge during full expiration, keeping the fingers elevated while sensing the systolic impulse and observing the motion imparted by the RV contraction. This technique is relatively insensitive in detecting subtle systolic movement and does not localize the impulse so derived.
2. A more refined method employs **several fingertips** applied simultaneously and in parallel in the third, fourth and fifth intercostal spaces during held exspiration. The free left hand is used for timing with the right carotid pulse as reference or by applying the stethoscope to the chest for the identification of the first and second heart sounds. This method of palpation not only permits detection of gentle RV systolic impulses but also localizes

the movements to the inflow portion (4th and 5th ICS) or infundibulum or outflow portion (3rd ICS). In infants, palpation along the left sternal border is achieved with the tip of a single finger during active breathing or during a very brief arrested respiration induced by pinching the nostrils while the infant sucks on a nipple or pacifier.

Causes of Parasternal Lift

RV Volume Overload
1. *Exaggerated motion* of the entire parasternal area (hyperdynamic impulse) usually reflects increased RV contractility due to augmented stroke volume as occurs in, atrial septal defect (ASD) or tricuspid regurgitation (TR).
2. *RV pressure overload:* A sustained left parasternal outward thrust reflect RV hypertrophy due to pressure overload, as in PAH or PS. Right ventricular failure (RVF) with reduced RV ejection produces a prolonged left parasternal impulse. When the RV is appreciably enlarged, it occupies the apex, displacing the left ventricle, which no longer makes contact with the chest wall and therefore imparts no precordial impulse. In this setting, RV systolic movement extends from the left sternal edge to the cardiac apex, which retracts. To confirm that the RV occupies the apex, observation of movement becomes important because lateral retraction is better seen than palpated.
3. *Left atrial impulse:* Significant mitral regurgitation (MR) may cause left atrial expansion during LV systole producing a sustained left parasternal impulse. Thus, at the bedside before the diagnosis of the RVF/RVH is suspected, it is necessary to exclude significant MR. In patients with RVH and RVF, however, a sustained epigastric impulse is appreciated. The systolic bulging of the left atrium (LA), which is transmitted through the RV, commences and terminates after the LV thrust. Movement imparted by the systolic expansion of the LA can be appreciated by placing the index finger of one hand at the LV apex and the index finger of the other in the left parasternal region in the third intercostal space; the movement of the latter finger begins and ends slightly later than that of the former.

A giant left atrium may extend well in to the right hemithorax, so mitral regurgitation can cause late systolic movement of the lower right anterior chest, occasionally as far as the right anterior axillary line. When MR occurs in the presence of a dilated left atrial appendage, an impulse is palpated and often seen in the third left interspace because the appendage is border forming at that site.

Dressler's Grading of Parasternal lift

Grade 1: Faintly felt
Grade 2: Felt, seen, but can be obliterated with pressure
Grade 3: Cannot be obliterated with pressure.

EPIGASTRIC IMPULSE

In the subxiphoid region, which allows palpation of the right ventricle, should be examined with the tip of the **index finger during held inspiration**. This technique is particularly useful in patients with an increased anteroposterior diameter, COPD, obesity, or a muscular chest, when RV enlargement is suspected, but a parasternal impulse cannot be felt. With the hand flattened the index finger should be pressed just under the rib cage and up toward the left shoulder. The examiner should be careful to differentiate the downward - directed motion of the enlarged RV from the anterior pulsations of the abdominal aorta, which can often be felt in the epigastrium. Palpable RV diastolic events are often best detected with this approach.

PA Impulse

Pulmonary artery: The main pulmonary trunk (MPA) is border forming in the second left interspace. The impulse is often better seen than palpated, especially when observed during full held expiration with the site marked with an 'X'. In thin patients, especially with decreased anteroposterior chest dimensions, a normal pulmonary trunk sometimes transmits a visible and palpable impulse to the 2nd left interspace prominent during full held expiration. PAH or increase in pulmonary blood flow (PBF) produce a prominent systolic pulsation of the pulmonary trunk in the second intercostal space just left of the sternum. This may be associated with a palpable shock synchronous with the second heart sound, reflecting forceful closure of the pulmonary valve.

AORTIC Impulse

Aorta: Sternoclavicular joint pulsations are rarely visible. They are generally subtle, and are best sensed by relatively firm pressure with two apposed fingertips, which fix the point under examination. Enlargement or aneurysm of the ascending aorta or the aortic arch may cause visible or palpable systolic pulsation of the right or left sternoclavicular joint and may also cause a systolic impulse in the suprasternal notch or in the first or second right intercostal spaces.

However, the most common cause of the right supraclavicular pulsation is a kinked, tortuous right carotid artery. An abnormal pulsation of a sternoclavicular joint in patients with chest pain may be a early clue to diagnosis of aortic dissection. A slight pulsation in the right sternoclavicular area may suggest a right sided aortic arch in patients with cyanotic heart disease.

Rarely, late systolic anterior movement of the sternum (and of the contiguous left parasternal area) is caused by a large, pulsatile descending aortic aneurysm as it physically moves the heart forward during ventricular systole. If this sign is suspected, a synchronous late systolic movement should be sought in the posterior thorax to the left of the vertebral column.

THRILLS

Definition: Thrills are palpable vibrations from the murmurs or bruit, ordinarily associated with grade 4/6 murmur or louder.

The flat of the hand or the finger tips usually best appreciate thrills, which are vibratory sensation that are palpable manifestations of loud, harsh murmurs having low to medium frequency components. Thrills are most readily characterized according to their *timing* in the cardiac cycle (systolic, diastolic or continuous), their *location*, their direction of *radiation*, and their *duration*. High pitched murmurs such as those produced by valvular regurgitation, even when loud are not usually associated with thrills.

Systolic thrills at the right or left base as in AS or PS can be palpated with the patient supine at 30–45 degrees, or still better with the patient sitting and leaning forward during full held expiration. When the thrill is prominent and widespread, application of the entire palm of the hand is sometimes helpful in sensing the direction of radiation of the aortic stenotic thrill upward and to the right, and radiation of the pulmonic stenotic thrill upward and to the left.

Thrills may be felt at the apex in MR and HOCM, lower left sternal border in VSD. It is useful to localize the site of maximum intensity of a left parasternal systolic thrill. Maximum intensity in the second intercostal space occurs in pulmonic valve stenosis, in the third intercostal space in infundibular pulmonic stenosis, and in the fourth or fifth intercostal space with ventricular septal defect (VSD). Two or three fingers can be applied simultaneously in the 2nd, 3rd and 4th or 4th, 5th and 6th interspaces. Most systolic thrills are better identified during expiration, but the thrill of tricuspid regurgitation is better sensed or may appear only during inspiration.

An **early diastolic left parasternal thrill** is more likely to accompany aortic regurgitation (AR), less likely the Graham Steel murmur of high pressure PR, because the latter is usually grade 3 or less. The best technique for eliciting these left parasternal high frequency early diastolic thrills is by applying the distal metacarpals or fingertips at the left sternal edge with the patient first supine at 30–45 degrees and then sitting and leaning forward during full held expiration. When the diastolic thrill of AR is better detected at the right sternal edge, the cause is likely to be a dilated aortic root, as in Marfan syndrome.

Systolic and diastolic **thrills at the apex** are best assessed during held expiration with the patient in a partial left lateral decubitus position. An intense systolic thrill of MR commonly radiates into the axilla, sometimes to the left sternal edge, to the base, and even into the neck.

A diastolic thrill occasionally may be felt at the apex in the lateral decubitus position in MS. Equivocal thrills often become more pronounced when the patient voluntarily coughs briskly, a maneuver that transiently increases the heart rate and mitral flow.

Gently placing a fingertip in the suprasternal notch will allow detection of thrills in patients with aortic valve stenosis, pulmonary valve stenosis, aortic regurgitation, PDA, or coarctation of aorta. In these lesions, a thrill may also be palpable over the carotid arteries.

Stenotic RV-PA conduits may produce a thrill. These are usually felt along the left sternal border.

PALPABLE SOUNDS

Prominent S1 (mitral component): It may be sometimes palpable over the LV impulse in the left lateral decubitus position during held expiration in thin, slightly built subjects, especially if the PR interval is short and cardiac rate rapid. Palpation is best accomplished by relatively firm pressure of a fingertip. In rheumatic mitral stenosis with mobile anterior leaflet, a loud first heart is often more readily palpable than accompanying LV impulse.

Aortic component (A2): Loud aortic valve closure sounds may be audible. This is often palpable in the second right interspace in the presence of simple systemic hypertension. This is also palpable when the aortic root is dilated and the pulmonary trunk small (as in severe TOF or pulmonary atresia) or when the aortic root is anterior to the pulmonary trunk as in complete transposition of the great arteries.

Pulmonary component (P2): The pulmonic component of the second heart sound is palpated in the second left interspace in patients with pulmonary arterial hypertension (PAH), although dilatation of the pulmonary trunk with normal pulmonary arterial pressure occasionally renders the pulmonic component palpable. In some normal children and adolescents and in thin subjects with decreased anteroposterior chest dimensions, a normal pulmonic component of the second heart sound is occasionally palpated as a gentle tap. Palpation is enhanced when a fingertip is applied between the ribs in the 2nd LICS with moderate pressure during held expiration. Pressure at the same site with the distal metacarpal is also useful. A very loud pulmonic component transmits widely to the mid and lower left sternal edge, right base, and apex, especially when the RV occupies the apex.

Aortic ejection sounds: In congenital aortic stenosis (AS), it may be more readily palpated over the LV impulse than in the second right interspace, and therefore must be distinguished from a loud first heart sound. A normal PR interval and a relatively slow heart rate assist in this distinction. Aortic ejection sounds that originate within a dilated aortic root (in contrast to origin in the valve itself) are better palpated at the right base over the site of systolic movement of the dilated aorta. Palpation is accomplished at this site by moderately firm pressure of a fingertip applied during held expiration or by firmly applying the distal metacarpals.

Pulmonary ejection sound: This may be palpable in the second left intercostal space and are sometimes sensed only during normal expiration, diminishing or vanishing altogether during normal inspiration.

Presystolic pulsation: (usually accompanying a S4) may be palpable. It is best palpated during exhalation, when the patient is in left lateral decubitus position with light pressure of fingertips over the apex. It can be confirmed by observing the motion of an X mark over the left ventricular impulse. It can be enhanced by sustained handgrip. Audibility of the S4 does not correlate with palpability; presystolic expansion may be detectable when the S4 is quite soft. Occasionally one may not hear an S4, when it is clearly palpable, because of the extremely low frequency vibrations of the diastolic filling event, usually less than 50 cycles per second.

Diastolic heart beat: The precordial diastolic movement in chronic constrictive pericarditis has been called the "diastolic heart beat". This movement coincides with rapid diastolic flow into the constricted ventricles (left and right) and is synchronous with the brisk Y trough of JVP.

Opening snap: The most common early diastolic sound amenable to palpation because of intensity per se is the opening snap of mitral stenosis. The sound is palpable over the left ventricular impulse, but when loud, radiates to the lower left sternal edge.

Tumor plop: A relatively rare palpable early diastolic sound—the "tumor plop"—is generated during abrupt deceleration of a mobile, pedunculated right or left atrial myxoma as the tumor seats within the tricuspid or mitral orifice.

CHAPTER 6

First Heart Sound

Oomen K George, Bobby John

CHAPTER OUTLINE

- First Heart Sound
- Components of First Heart Sound
- Theories of Generation of First Heart Sound
- Intensity of S1
- Pathological First Heart Sound
- Split First Heart Sound

Sound is defined as vibrations that are audible because of their appropriate amplitude and frequency. Human ear is capable of detecting sound vibrations between 30 and 18000 Hz. Most cardiovascular sounds and murmurs are in the frequency range between 30 and 1000 Hz, which is below the optimal range of hearing. Human ear can distinguish sounds occurring 20 msec apart.

FIRST HEART SOUND

The first heart sound (S1) signals the onset of LV contraction which occurs 50-60 msec after the electrical initiation of LV systole, frequency ranges from 100 to 120 Hz, occurs with the upstroke of the carotid impulse.

COMPONENTS OF FIRST HEART SOUND

1. Small low frequency vibrations—muscular in origin.
2. Large high frequency vibrations that are easily audible, related to closure of mitral valve (M1).
3. Second high frequency component related to tricuspid valve closure (T1); occurs 20-30 msec after M1.
4. Small low frequency vibrations that coincide with the accelerated flow of blood into the great vessels.

THEORIES OF GENERATION OF FIRST HEART SOUND

1. Luisada—due to prominent tensing of the LV walls, septum, and mitral valve apparatus, which produces a sound transient. Luisada thought that the second major vibration of S1 is due to the opening of aortic valve. But

this also has been proven to be related to tricuspid valve closure. M1 coincides with the down stroke of the left atrial c wave and T1 with that of the right atrial c wave.
2. Leatham—due to sudden tensing of closed mitral valve leaflets, which leads to sudden deceleration of blood, setting the surrounding cardiac structures into vibration.

INTENSITY OF S1

The primary factors determining this are as follows:
1. *Integrity* of valve closure-inadequate coaptation leads to a soft S1 as in MR.
2. *Mobility of the valve*: calcified valve leads to a soft S1.
3. *Velocity of valve closure* - the most important factor. This is determined by the timing of mitral valve closure in relation to the left ventricular pressure rise in early systole. At short PR intervals (30–70 msec), the mitral valve leaflets are maximally separated by atrial contraction at the onset of LV contraction and the mitral valve close at a high velocity with a large excursion resulting in a loud S1.
4. *Status of ventricular contraction*: This relates to the rate of pressure development in the LV. Exercise, adrenaline, high output states often associated with tachycardia leads to increase in the intensity of S1, decreased in myxedema, cardiomyopathy and acute myocardial infarction.
5. *Transmission characteristics* of the thoracic cavity and the chest wall: obesity, emphysema, large pleural or pericardial effusions decrease the intensity of S1.
6. *Physical characteristics of the vibrating structures*: Myocardial Infarction and ischemia induced by pacing also has shown to decrease the intensity of S1.

Beat-to-beat variation in the intensity of S1: It is seen in:
1. Complete heart block with AV dissociation—the loud intermittent cannon sound in this condition is called bruit de cannon.
2. Mobitz type 1 heart block
3. VT with AV dissociation
4. Atrial fibrillation and mitral stenosis:
    – Type I: In mild MS, less tendency of the S1 to become louder after long diastoles
    – Type II: In tight calcified MS, the M1 depends entirely on preceding and pre preceding RR intervals (Starling and postextrasystolic potentiation effect). Here the S1 becomes louder in proportion to the length of the previous diastole
    – Type III: In moderate stenosis, the loudness varies inversely with the duration of the previous diastole.
5. Pulse paradoxus—S1 gets softer on inspiration.

LOUD FIRST HEART SOUND

First sound is said to be loud when it is louder than the second heart sound in the right second intercostal space.

Causes of Loud S1

1. Mitral valve obstruction—MS with mobile anterior leaflet, LA myxoma.
2. Tachycardia or hyperkinetic states.
3. Short PR interval—less than 160 msec (Also if > 360 msec).
4. Hypertension.
5. Hyperthyroidism.
6. Short cycle lengths in atrial fibrillation.
7. L to R shunts PDA, VSD.
8. ASD.
9. Tricuspid valve obstruction—TS, RA myxoma.
10. Ebstein's anomaly.
11. Thin chest wall.
12. Holosystolic MVP—due to the increased amplitude of leaflet excursion with prolapse beyond the line of closure or due to the summation of a normal M1 and early ejection click. In the more common variety of middle or late systolic prolapse, S1 is normal; If soft, it indicates a flail mitral leaflet.

Mitral Stenosis

In MS, the increased left atrial pressure delays the time of pressure cross over between the LA and the LV. As a result M1 occurs later and at a much higher than normal LV pressure, at a time when there is more rapid rate of development of LV pressure rise. Secondly, the greater than normal excursion of the mitral valve in mitral stenosis leads to the increased velocity of mitral valve closure causing a loud S1.

SOFT FIRST HEART SOUND

First heart sound is said to be soft when it is softer than S2 at the apex or left sternal border.

Causes of Soft S1

1. Long PR interval—more than 200 msec.
2. Depressed LV contractility.
3. Thick chest wall.
4. Emphysema.
5. Pericardial effusion.
6. MR.
7. Depressed LV contractility.
8. Ectopic beats.

9. Flail mitral leaflet.
10. LBBB.
11. Hemodynamically significant AS.

LBBB: S1 is soft because of the delay in ventricular contraction, degree of LV dysfunction, presence of concomitant first degree heart block and the presence a noncompliant LV leading to preclosure of the mitral valve.

SPLIT S1

Normally M1 precedes T1, is synchronous or is narrowly split, (20 to 40 msec apart), heard exclusively in the left lower sternal border.

Pathological split: This occurs when T1 is more separated from M1. It is seen in the following conditions:
- RBBB
- LV pacing
- WPW syndrome
- Tricuspid Stenosis
- Ebstein's anomaly—SAIL SOUND is the exaggerated T1, which is widely separated from M1, pathognomonic.

Windsock Sound: This is a widely split S1 associated with sudden slapping motion of a ventricular septal aneurysm into RV or occurs in a VSD that is closing.

Reverse splitting of S1

This occurs when M1 preceds T1. It is seen in the following conditions:
- LA myxoma
- Mitral Stenosis
- LBBB
- RV pacing.

Hemodynamic Correlation of S1

- Mitral component of S1 occurs at the downstroke of the left atrial C wave
- It occurs after 30 msec of LV—LA pressure cross over. (mitral flow inertia is the reason).

CHAPTER 7

Second Heart Sound

Oomen K George, Bobby John

CHAPTER OUTLINE

- Theories of Generation of Second Heart Sound
- Abnormal Intensity of Second Heart Sound
- Split Second Heart Sound
- Paradoxical Split
- Reverse Paradoxical Split
- Single Second Heart Sound

The second heart sound was labeled by Leatham as the key to auscultation of the heart, is of frequency 120–150 Hz, and coincides with the down stroke of the carotid pulse. Two components, the earlier one is due to aortic valve closure (A2) and the later one is due to pulmonary valve closure (P2)

THEORIES OF GENERATION OF SECOND HEART SOUND

Second heart sound occurs as a result of sudden deceleration of retrograde blood flow in the aorta and pulmonary artery, which sets the cardiohemic system into vibration causing the sounds.

HANG OUT INTERVAL

Though the right and left ventricular systoles are equal in duration, the pulmonary artery incisura is delayed in relation to the aortic incisura, primarily due to a larger interval separating the pulmonary artery incisura from the RV pressure compared with the same left-sided event. This interval is termed as the hang out interval. Its duration is a reflection of the impedance of the vascular bed that receives the blood.

ABNORMALITIES OF S2 INTENSITY

A loud aortic component (A2) occurs when there is increased flow and or pressure in the aorta. Root dilatation also can increase intensity of A2.

The decrease in intensity of A2 is due to lack of apposition of leaflets and decrease in arterial diastolic pressure (Table 1).

Table 1
Increased and decreased intensity of A2

Increased intensity of A2	Decreased intensity of A2
1. Systemic hypertension (drum like or tambour S2)	1. Aortic Regurgitation
2. Coarctation of aorta	2. Valvar and Supravalvar aortic stenosis
3. Ascending aortic aneurysm	
4. Relative anterior placement of the aorta Tetrology of Fallot Transposition of Great arteries	

Increased Intensity of P2

Normally P2 is not audible at the apex. If P2 is louder than A2 in 2nd left intercostal space (ICS) or if it is audible at the apex, it is said to be loud. A loud P2 indicates elevated pulmonary pressures except in ASD where because of the enlarged right ventricle, P2 may be audible at the apex even in the absence of elevated PA pressures. However, if P2 is very loud or it increases after mild exercise, the presence of an ASD with pulmonary hypertension (PH) and elevated pulmonary vascular resistance PVR should be suspected (Table 1).

Soft P2

1. Pulmonary stenosis.
2. PR due absent pulmonary valve (In PR due to PAH P2 may be loud).
3. TOF. P2 is inaudible except in milder cases where delayed P2 may be heard.

Masking: A loud A2 or an early opening snap may mask P2. So also long holosystolic murmurs (VSD, PS, MR). Soft A2 with loud P2 is heard in the setting of a low cardiac output like in massive pulmonary embolism.

SPLITTING OF S2

Splitting of S2 refers to the presence of two audible components at the end of expiration. This indicates an interval of at least 30–40 msec between the two sounds. This is enhanced when the subject is upright because RV systole shortens more than LV systole on standing. When there is no detectable change in the S2 interval, the split is considered fixed.

Mechanism of Splitting

Traditional explanation: Increased venous return during inspiration leads to prolongation of the RV systole, while a concomitant decrease in venous return to left heart leads to shortened LV systole. Immediate inspiratory increase in RV stroke volume is followed 1–3 cardiac cycles by a similar increase in stroke volume of the left ventricle and an increase in the LV ejection time, which occurs in expiration.

Recent explanation: The physiologic splitting of S2 in normal subjects is most probably due to an inspiratory decrease in the impedance of the pulmonary bed rather than due to prolongation of RV systole. When the normal impedance characteristics of this bed are lost as in pulmonary hypertension, inspiratory augmentation must occur primarily via increases in RV systole.

Types of S2 Splitting

1. Wide split.
2. Fixed split.
3. Paradoxical split.

Wide Split S2 (Also Called As Persistent Split)

If A2–P2 separation is appreciated in semi-recumbent, sitting or standing position during expiration, wide splitting of S2 should be suspected. For this the interval should be more than 0.03 sec.

Causes of audible expiratory splitting of S2 - Increased q-p2 (prolonged RV systole)

Hemodynamic causes

1. Pulmonary stenosis with intact septum : A2-P2 Delay >100 msec indicates an RV-PA gradient of 100 mm Hg when there is no infundibular stenosis.
2. Massive pulmonary embolism.
3. Pulmonary hypertension with RV failure.
4. ASD.
5. Idiopathic dilatation of PA.
6. Severe biventricular heart failure.

Electrical causes

1. Complete RBBB.
2. PVCs of LV origin/LV epicardial pacing.
3. WPW syndrome with LV preexcitation.

Decreased q-a2 interval (shortened LV systole)

1. Mitral regurgitation.
2. VSD.
3. Pericardial tamponade - LV filling may markedly decrease during inspiration unlike that of RV.
4. LA myxoma.
5. Constrictive pericarditis.

Other Causes

1. Pectus excavatum.
2. Straight back syndrome.
3. Occasionally normal children.

FIXED SPLITTING

1. When right or left ventricular *stroke volume does not change* during inspiration such as in RV failure, acute and chronic pulmonary embolism and severe PH.
2. When there is *similar degree of alteration* in LV and RV filling—ASD, VSD with markedly elevated PVR because of the comparable delay in both the chambers.

REVERSED OR PARADOXICAL SPLITTING

Reversed splitting occurs when S2 is maximally split on expiration and narrows or fuses during inspiration. This is generally due to delay in A2.

There are 3 types of Paradoxical Spliting.
Type I
Type II
Type III.

Type I Paradoxical Splitting (The Most Common)

During expiration, prolonged LV systole causes A2 to follow P2. With inspiration, the Q-P2 increases normally but Q-A2 is unchanged or shortens. The two components of S2 occur so close that the ear appreciates only a single second sound (Fig. 1).

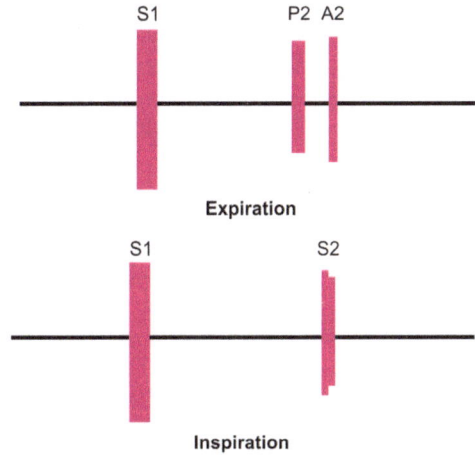

Figure 1 Type I paradoxical splitting

Type II Paradoxical Splitting

In lesser degrees of Q-A2 delay, or with a wide inspiratory lengthening of Q-P2 delay, inspiration may still result in normal A2-P2 relationship and audible splitting, although S2 reversal occurs in inspiration (Fig. 2).

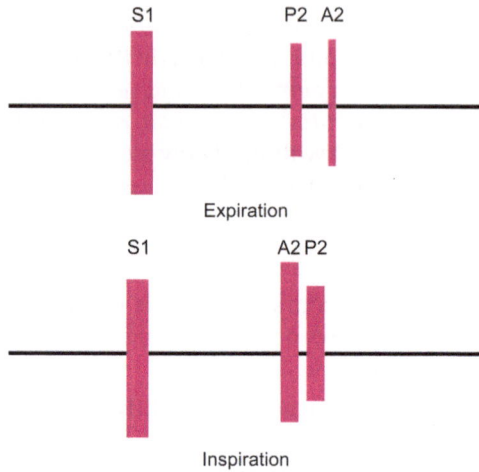

Figure 2 Type II paradoxical splitting

Type III Paradoxical Splitting

If both inspiratory and expiratory separation of A2 and P2 are 20 msec or less apart, S2 will be heard as a single sound or fused in both phases of respiration, even though A2 follows P2 in expiration (Fig. 3).

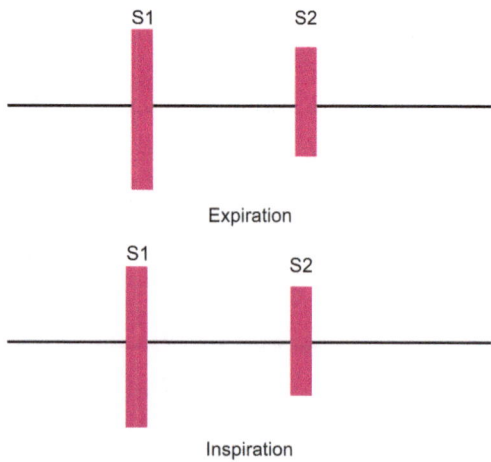

Figure 3 Type III paradoxical splitting

Causes

Delayed aortic closure
a. Delayed electrical activation of the LV:
   1. Complete LBBB-most common causes: due to delayed activation of LV and prolonged isovolumetric contraction time, RV paced beats, RV ectopics.
   2. Type B WPW syndrome.
   3. Hypertensive heart disease.
   4. Chronic IHD.
   5. Angina Pectoris.
   6. LVOT obstruction.
   7. Severe AS (may be due to increased hang out interval also).
b. Decreased impedance of systemic vascular bed
   1. Post-stenotic dilatation of the aorta secondary to AS or AR.
   2. PDA.
   3. Chronic AR.

Pseudoparadoxical Splitting

In patients with large chests or COPD, inspiration may cause an artifactual muffling or disappearance of P2 due to interposition of the expanded lung between the stethoscope and aorta, which may be mistaken for paradoxical splitting.

Narrow Physiologic Splitting

The splitting interval is less than 30 msec, but both components are easily heard due to the increased intensity and the high frequency composition of P2. It occurs in severe pulmonary hypertension without RV failure.

SINGLE S2

I. Absence of either component of S2 or fusion of A2 P2 without inspiratory split gives rise to single S2
1. Absent P2.
2. Truncus arteriosus.
3. TOF.
4. Severe semilunar valve stenosis.
5. Pulmonary atresia.
6. Most cases of tricuspid atresia.

II. Fusion of A2 and P2

1. Eisenmenger VSD.
2. Single ventricle.

III. Apparently Single S2 (Due to Inaudibility of P2)

1. Emphysema.
2. Obesity.
3. Pericardial effusion.

The cause/type of single S2 should be determined by the accompanying clinical features.

Third Heart Sound

Oomen K George, Bobby John

CHAPTER OUTLINE

- Mechanism of Production
- Left Ventricular S3
- Right Ventricular S3
- Prognostic Importance
- Maneuvers to Augment S3
- Causes of S3
- Causes of Right Ventricular S3
- Differentiation from Opening Snap

MECHANISM OF PRODUCTION OF THIRD HEART SOUND

Impact Theory (Most Accepted)

Rapid ventricular filling occurs early in diastole when atrioventricular valves are open completely. If the ventricles resist this rapid inflow, vibratory activity may result. If this vibratory activity becomes sufficiently intense to be transmitted from the ventricles to the chest wall, a third heart sound will be produced.

Ventricular Theory by Leatham

Third heart sound (S3) occurs due to sudden cessation of filling of blood from the atria to the ventricles resulting in distension and vibration of the ventricular wall, papillary muscles and chordae.

Valvular Theory

Onset of S3 occurs due to sudden limitation of longitudinal expansion of the LV wall during early diastole. Normal S3 occurs due to sudden limitation of longitudinal expansion of the LV wall during early diastolic filling. Abnormal S3 is generated by altered physical properties of the recipient ventricle and/or an increase in the rate and volume of atrioventricular flow during the rapid filling phase of the cardiac cycle.

S3 implies rapid inflow and denies obstructive lesion at the appropriate atrioventricular valve. It is a low-pitched sound heard in early diastole. It is often better palpable than audible. S3 may be physiological or pathological. S3 is heard in majority of children, 50% of young adults, occasionally in middle aged and rarely in the elderly. S3 may be heard in either or both the ventricles and is heard best with the bell of the stethoscope with light pressure applied to form a skin seal.

CLINICAL

- **Left ventricular S3** is heard best at the area of the apical impulse with patient lying in the left lateral position with patient exhaling
- **Right ventricular S3** is heard best at the lower left sternal border at the fourth or fifth interspace and also the epigastrium. Intensity of RV S3 increases with inspiration. S3 becomes fainter when patient sits or stands. It waxes and wanes with normal phases of respiration. At times instead of being detected with every beat, they can be heard during sinus tachycardia. S3 coincides with the latter portion of the descending limb of the "v" wave of the JVP. It coincides with the Y descent of the atrial pressure pulse. It is heard 0.13 – 0.18 sec after A2
- In constrictive pericarditis the additional heart sound is loud and of higher frequency due to calcification of the pericardium; and heard early, i.e. 0.10 – 0.12 seconds after A2. This is also called as the "pericardial knock".

Gallop rhythm: This is an auscultatory phenomenon in which a tripling or quadrupling of heart sounds resembles the canter of a horse. Addition of S3 or S4 forms the **triple rhythm**. **Quadruple rhythm** both S3 and S4 are present. **Diastolic gallop** is the cadence produced by S3 in heart failure. It is one of the earliest clinical findings of cardiac failure. When S3 and S4 occur in close proximity to each other a diastolic rumble can be produced, which is more common in tachycardia.

- **Third heart sound and cardiac failure:** Pulsus alternans is almost always associated with S3. It can also prognosticate. Life expectancy after ventricular gallop is 4–5 years. Louder the gallop, poorer the prognosis and worse if it persists despite medical management
- **Physiological S3:** This occurs at the same timing. It waxes and wanes in intensity with respiration. Physiological S3 is rarely heard in those above 30 years of age
- **Maneuvers to augment the audibility of S3**
  - **Exercise:** S3 audibility is improved by isotonic exercise that augments venous return and mid diastolic atrioventricular flow like walking, climbing stairs, and performing number of sit ups
  - **Tachycardia:** It is also augmented due to tachycardia produced by having the patient cough 5–6 times

- **Leg Raising:** Increasing venous return by passive leg raising can augment S3
- **Post-VPC:** If patient has S3 and ventricular premature beats, the intensity of the gallop sound is accentuated for a few beats following the VPCs. This is called the post extrasystolic accentuation. S3 can be heard in normal hearts after extrasystoles—this is benign. Gallop rhythm heard temporarily after cessation of tachycardia as in atrial tachycardia usually benign.

CAUSES OF LV S3

a. *Conditions which increase cardiac output*
- Anemia
- Mitral regurgitation
- Hyperthyroidism
- VSD
- Aortic regurgitation
- PDA
- Exercise
- Pregnancy

b. *Left Ventricular Failure*

CAUSES OF RV S3

- ASD
- Right Heart Failure
- Severe TR
- Cor pulmonale
- Massive pulmonary embolism
- Loudest S3 is heard in constrictive pericarditis

RV S3 is localized to left lower sternal border and increases with inspiration, whereas LV S3 is localized to the apex.

DIFFERENTIATION OF S3 AND OPENING SNAP

Opening snap occurs earlier. It is sharper, louder and heard best at left border of lower sternum (Table 1).

Table 1

Differentiation of S3 and opening snap

	S3	Opening snap
Site	Apex	Just internal to Apex
Radiation	None	All over precardium
Pitch	Low pitch	High pitch
Timing	0.13 seconds or more	0.08 seconds to 0.12 seconds

CHAPTER 9

Fourth Heart Sound

Oomen K George, Bobby John

CHAPTER OUTLINE

- Definition
- Mechanism of Production
- Left Ventricular S4
- Right Ventricular S4
- Temporal Sequence
- Associated Disease Conditions
- Differentiation from Two components of S1
- Summation Gallop

DEFINITION

Sound generated during atrial filling phase within the recipient ventricle is called as the fourth heart sound (S4). It is also called as atrial or ***presystolic gallop*** or triple rhythm. It is a low-pitched sound that varies considerably in intensity and heard better with the bell of the stethoscope with light pressure applied to form a skin seal.

MECHANISM OF PRODUCTION

It is caused by increase in stiffness of the ventricles; atrial contraction as a consequence produces sudden increases in pressure in the ventricle, rather than the ventricle increasing in its volume to accommodate the extra-blood delivered by atrial systole.

Left Ventricular S4

LV S4 is heard well at the point of maximal LV impulse with the patient in the left lateral position. It may be palpable in this position. It may even be seen by examining the movement of a lightweight pencil held over the point of maximal impulse. It can be induced or augmented when resistance of LV discharge is increased by sustained handgrip especially in presence of coronary artery disease.

Right Ventricular S4

RV S4 is heard at the lower left sternal border or the subxiphoid region or the right external jugular vein with the patient in the supine position. Inspiration causes an increase in the right atrial blood flow, which is converted into an inspiratory augmentation of both mid diastolic and presystolic filling and hence RV S4 is louder during inspiration. Fourth heart sound precedes S1.

Temporal Sequence

The interval between the presystolic sound and S1 is variable, being longer or shorter according to whether the ventricle concerned is under greater or less strain respectively. S4 occurs with peak of *a* wave in apex cardiogram. LV S4 is temporally related to "a" point of the mitral valve motion. As LV function improves, the gallop sound gradually merges into the first sound. S4 disappears when coordinated atrial contraction ceases, as in atrial fibrillation. S4 is an event of ventricular filling, so obstruction of an AV valve, by impending ventricular flow, removes one of the prime preconditions for the generation of these filling sounds, therefore presence of S3 or S4 implies an unobstructed (or relatively unobstructed) AV orifice on the side of the heart in which it originates. S4 does not occur with mitral stenosis or tricuspid stenosis.

FOURTH HEART SOUND IN DISEASE CONDITIONS

1. Atrioventricular Block

S4 may be heard in Ist, IInd or IIIrd degree AV block. With normal PQ (PR) interval an atrial gallop is not detected, since the atrial gallop sound occurs at the specified interval from the atrial contraction (i.e at an interval of 0.16 s after beginning of the P wave on the ECG). Although a faint sound may normally be present, it is merged with the S1. When *PR interval is prolonged* i.e. 0.22–0.26 sec, an atrial gallop sound is heard in addition to faint S1. These two findings provided a bedside clue to first-degree heart block.

With *second-degree heart block*, the atrial gallop is easily heard. In patients with constant 2:1 AV block, the atrial sound often occurs at the approximate timing of the normal S3 of ventricular diastole, resulting in prominent sound in early part of diastole.

In *complete heart block*, atrial gallop sounds are frequently heard. When atria and ventricles contract independently, S4 or summation sounds occur randomly in diastole because relationship between P wave and QRS of ECG is random. Careful auscultation in a quite room is necessary to detect these sounds, which resemble faint footsteps on a carpet.

2. Coronary Artery Disease

It is unusual not to hear a faint S4 in a patient who has had previous myocardial infarction (MI). S4 is louder during an episode of acute MI and pain or during initial phases of MI.

3. Cardiomyopathy

S4 heard in patients in sinus rhythm, becomes louder with exacerbation of symptoms.

4. Systemic Hypertension

It is heard especially in patients with persistent BP elevation.

5. Aortic Valve Disease

S4 in aortic stenosis occurs particularly in patients with higher degrees of obstruction. It correlates with systolic gradient of 70 mm Hg across the aortic valve or a LVEDP of 15 mm of Hg. It may also be heard in AR especially acute AR.

6. Age

Older patients may have S4 when there is minimal to moderate aortic valve gradient due to associated coronary artery disease. In patients under 40 years of age, there is better correlation of S4 with severity of AS.

7. Pulmonary Hypertension

More severe the obstruction, the more it is associated with atrial gallop (RV S4). It occurs when there is a change in ventricular compliance and increased resistance to filling.

8. Pulmonary Stenosis

It may also be heard with significant PS. RVS4 in PS indicates >100 mm Hg RVSP.

9. Bernheim Phenomenon

In patients with LV dysfunction there may be a conspicuous "a" wave in the JVP and atrial gallop best heard at the left sternal edge or epigastrium.

10. Other Conditions

S4 may also be heard when cardiac output and stroke volume are increased, as in thyrotoxicosis, anemia and large AV fistulas.

DIFFERENTIATION OF M1–T1 FROM S4–S1

The two components of S1 are similar in pitch although not in intensity and differ in pitch from a preceding S4. Selective pressure on the stethoscope enhances these differences.

Table 1
Causes of S4

Mechanism	Causes
Physiological	Nonaudible
Pathological – Decreased compliance	LVOT obstruction HCM Hypertension
Pathological – Ischemic heart disease	Angina, Acute MI, post-MI LV dysfunction
Rapid late diastolic filling	Anemia, thyrotoxicosis
Arrhythmia	AV block

SUMMATION GALLOP

In the presence of sinus tachycardia, atrial contraction may coincide with the rapid filling phase, to form the summation sound. Carotid sinus massage transiently slows the heart rate, so the diastolic sound or sounds can be assigned their proper timing (Table 1).

CHAPTER 10

Systolic and Diastolic Sounds

Oomen K George, Bobby John

CHAPTER OUTLINE

- Ejection Clicks
- Nonejection Clicks
- Opening Snap
- Pericardial Knock
- Prosthetic Valve Sounds

EJECTION CLICKS

Early Systolic Sounds

Aortic and pulmonary ejection sounds are the most common early systolic sounds. First heart sound (S1) occurs at the beginning of period of isometric contraction, an ejection sound occurs at the end of this period. The two sounds are separated by an interval of about 0.06–0.08 s. It occurs 0.12–0.14 s after Q wave of ECG. The ejection sounds may be aortic or pulmonary in origin. They are high frequency sounds, similar in frequency to S1.

Mechanism of Production

Valvar theory: Ejection sound coincides with the fully opened position of the relevant semilunar valve. It is caused by the abrupt cephalad doming of the valve.

Vascular theory: The origin of the sound within dilated arterial trunk guarded by a normal semilunar valve is assigned to opening movement of the leaflets that resonate in arterial or to the wall of the dilated artery.

Ejection sounds are more likely to occur with mild than in severe stenosis; or with mobile rather than immobile cusps.

Ejection Sounds and Phases of Respiration

Aortic ejection sounds do not vary with respiration except those that originate in the large biventricular aorta of tetralogy of Fallot with pulmonary atresia or truncus arteriosus.

Pulmonary ejection sounds decrease in intensity during normal inspiration.

Aortic Ejection Sound

It is sharp, brief and high-pitched; the intensity varying little with respiration. It is best heard at the apex and well transmitted over the precordium to the aortic area and even heard over the right carotid artery. It is found to occur with deformed aortic valve as in bicuspid aortic valve. A mobile valve is necessary to produce an ejection sound. It introduces the murmur in AS. The aortic ejection sound is coincident with the anacrotic notch on the upstroke of the aortic pressure curve.

Intensity of the ejection sound correlates with the mobility of the valve, but there is no correlation between the intensity and severity of stenosis. In mobile nonstenotic bicuspid valve, the ejection sound is not only loud but also widely separated from S1 due to prolonged excursion of the mobile valve. The ejection sound is absent when valve becomes calcified and less mobile.

Ejection sound may also occur with dilatation of ascending aorta and is heard in coarctation of aorta, systemic hypertension, atherosclerosis, idiopathic dilatation of ascending aorta and aortic root dilation associated with valvar AS.

It does not occur when obstruction is well proximal to the valve as in fibromuscular ring or HOCM; in these cases the ascending aorta is not dilated.

The ejection sound heard due to hypertension is usually less prominent than those due to valvular causes. This is not as widely transmitted and is confined to the upper right sternal border. It is said to occur due to tortuous sclerotic aortic root, tight noncompliant aortic root, and forceful LV ejection. Loudest ejection sound occurs with post stenotic dilatation in congenital AS.

Pulmonary Ejection Click

- It is confined to upper left sternal border
- Best heard in the pulmonary area or 3rd left ICS at the sternal edge
- The timing is earlier than aortic ejection sound, i.e. 0.09–0.11 s after Q wave on the ECG. It is a short, brief, rather metallic sound
- **Variable ejection click—increases in expiration** and decreases in inspiration.
  The variability is related to the elevated RVEDP in PS. With inspiration, there is increased venous return to RV and there is elevation of RVEDP beyond the PA diastolic pressure and so there is premature opening of the pulmonary valve in diastole itself. The cephalic excursion of the valve during ventricular systole is diminished, accounting for the inspiratory decrease in intensity of the ejection sound.

Pulmonary ES in Valvular PS

In very mild valvular pulmonary stenosis (PS) respiratory variation may be absent. In very severe valvular PS the excursion of the deformed valve and RV isovolumic contraction time decrease, resulting in migration of the ejection sound toward S1. Therefore, ejection sound of severe PS occurs slightly earlier with severe obstruction. The ejection sound is loudest with trivial or mild stenosis and may be absent when stenosis is severe. This is because when there is a severe PS, there is an increase in RVEDP when compared to that of PA, and the dome would then rise gently in late diastole.

Pulmonary ES in PH or IDPA

Pulmonary ES occurs with pulmonary root dilatation which could be either idiopathic or secondary to severe pulmonary hypertension. It may also occur in situations with increased pulmonary blood flow as in ASD with L to R shunt. A loud click may be heard even after repair of ASD. It can occur in post stenotic dilatation of the pulmonary artery (PA); but does not occur with infundibular stenosis where PA is not dilated. Ejection sound is early in PS due to low pressure in PA. In pulmonary arterial hypertension (PAH) it is relatively late, i.e. 0.06–0.08 s after M1 (Table 1).

NON-EJCTION CLICKS

This refers to sounds that arise from the Atrio Ventricular valves—either mitral or tricuspid valve.

Mitral Valve Prolapse

- It is usually due to systolic prolapse of the mitral valve leaflets, especially of the posterior leaflet
- The click occurs due to tensing of valves during systole.

Table 1
Aortic versus pulmonary ejection click

	Aortic click	Pulmonary click
Site	Aortic area	Pulmonary area
Conduction	Across the precardium	Left sternal border
Respiratory variation	Constant	Better heard in expiration
Ventricular dominance	LV	RV
Associated findings	Features of Aortic stenosis	Features of pulmonary stenosis or pulmonary hypertension

- It coincides with maximum systolic excursion of a prolapsed leaflet into the left atrium (LA) and is ascribed to sudden tensing of the redundant leaflets and elongated chordae tendinae
- It has a sharp, high frequency, clicking quality
- It may be an isolated finding occurring most often in middle to late systole, or there may be multiple clicks, presumably as a result of different areas of the large, redundant, scalloped mitral leaflets especially the posterior leaflet, prolapsing at different times. Click usually occurs at the time of maximal prolapse
- Special feature of MVP is the click's variability from examination to examination and from beat to beat. It may be replaced by late systolic clicks
- Dynamic auscultation of MVP (Table 2).

OPENING SNAP

- Opening of a normal atrioventricular valve (mitral or tricuspid valve) is almost always a silent event
- Opening snap (OS) is an early diastolic sound. It may be present in normal sinus rhythm and in atrial fibrillation (AF)
- It occurs at the maximal opening of the AV valve in early diastole
- It is a sharp, high pitched, brief sound
- It occurs 0.06–0.10 sec after aortic component of the second heart sound (A2)
- OS occurs at or shortly after the peak of 'v' wave of JVP
- The interval of S2 to OS represents the isovolumetric relaxation period of LV and is inversely proportional to the LA pressure. The higher the LA pressure, the shorter the interval between A2 and OS.

Table 2
MVP click and maneuvers

	Maneuvers	*S1 and click interval*
Decrease in Ventricular Size	Standing	Decreased
	Valsalva phase 2	
	Nitrates	
Increase in Ventricular size	Supine	Increased
	Squatting	
	Expiration	
	Phenylephrine	

Factors that influence timing of OS relative to A2
a. Rate of LA pressure decline
b. Level of LV pressure at the time of A2
c. Level of LA pressure

In older subjects with systolic hypertension, MS of appreciable severity can occur with or without a short A2-OS interval because the elevated LV systolic pressure takes longer to fall below the LA pressure. OS indicates that the mitral valve is mobile, at least its longer anterior leaflet. Therefore, OS is characteristic of a stenotic but still pliable valve, and may occasionally occur when there is swift opening of nonstenotic valve, such as in torrential flow in severe mitral regurgitation (MR) and ASD. A functional OS may be heard in large VSD, thyrotoxicosis and Tricuspid Atresia with large ASD, second and third degree heart block and TOF after a BT shunt (Table 3).

Table 3
Causes of opening snap

1.	Mitral stenosis
2.	Tricuspid stenosis
3.	Severe Mitral regurgitation
4.	Atrial septal defect
5.	Large ventricular septal defect
6.	Tricuspid atresia with large ASD
7.	BT shunt
8.	Tetrology of Fallot
9.	Second and third degree heart block

S2 - OS Interval

Narrow 2 – OS interval Less than 0.08 sec	Long more than 0.10
MS tight	MS mild
Tachycardia	Hypertension – aortic systolic bp > 130, 2-OS is unreliable
	Bradycardia
	Poor LV function
	Aortic regurgitation
	Low LA pressure due to large LA

A short 2-OS interval is more reliable than large 2-OS interval because there are several reasons for a long interval.

S2-OS Interval and Its Relationship to the Severity of Mitral Stenosis

Severity	S2-OS interval
Mild	100–120 msec
Moderate	80–100 msec
Severe	<80 msec

Causes of Soft OS in Mitral Stenosis

1. Calcific valve
2. Low flow
3. AR severe

Differentiation Of S3 and Opening Snap

- S3 is low pitched sound and occurs 0.12 s after A2. It is a localized to one area and not conducted.
- OS is a high pitched sound and occurs earlier in timing. Best heard just internal to apex and well heard all over the precardium.

PERICARDIAL KNOCK

- The most impressive abnormality during auscultation in patients with constrictive pericarditis is the diastolic pericardial knock, an early diastolic sound that is often heard along the left sternal border. The same sound is heard infrequently in sub acute constrictive pericarditis of the fibroelastic variety, but not heard in pure cardiac tamponade
- The pericardial knock usually occurs 0.09 to 0.12 s after A2
- Timing to the sudden cessation of ventricular filling and the premature diastolic plateau of the diastolic ventricular volume curve (Table 4).

Table 4
Differentiation of P2 and OS

	Opening snap (OS)	P2
Site	Maximum intensity at apex	Maximum intensity at 2nd left intercostal space
Timing	Occurs later than P2	Occurs earlier than OS
Respiration	During inspiration A2-OS interval widens and three sequential sounds (A2, P2, OS)	Inspiration separates A2 and P2

PROSTHETIC VALVE SOUNDS

Caged Ball and disk valve prostheses produce an opening and a closing sound. The sound produced by caged ball valve is louder than the normal heart sound and is of different quality. At times more than one sound of a normally functioning valve is made at the time of opening and/or closing. A series of rattles or clicks is characteristic of a non-functional valve. Bioprosthetic valves do not produce an audible opening sound in the aortic position, but a distinct, well-defined closing sound may be produced (Tables 5 and 6).

Table 5
Differentiation of sounds around S1

Feature	Split S1	S1-EC	S1 – NEC	S4 – S4
Site of sound	Tricuspid area	Base	Apex	Apex
Audibility	Localized	Widely audible	Widely audible	Localized
Character	Low frequency	High, frequency sharp	High frequency sharp clicking	Low frequency
Palpation	Not palpable	Not palpable	Not palpable	Palpable
Maneuvers	Best heard during inspiration	No change in aortic ejection	NEC- louder and becomes earlier with standing	Isometric handgrip increases surgery

Table 6
Differentiation of sounds around S2

Feature	Split S2	S2-OS	S2 – S3	NEC-S2
Site of sound	Pulmonary area	Medial to apex	Apex	Apex
Audibility	Localized	Widely audible	Localized	Variable
Character	High pitch	High pitch	Low pitch	High pitch
Palpation	P2 may be palpable in PH	Not palpable	Palpable	Not palpable
Manuvers	Inspiration prolongs P2	No change with inspiration	LVS3- better heard in expiration. RVS3 -better heard in inspiration	Change with posture

Carabello. Modern management of mitral stenosis. Circulation. 2005; 112:432-8

CHAPTER 11

Diastolic Murmurs

Oomen K George, Bobby John

CHAPTER OUTLINE

- Definition
- Classification
- Mechanism
- Early Diastolic Murmurs
- Mid-diastolic Murmurs
- Late Diastolic or Presystolic Murmurs
- Innocent Diastolic Murmurs
- Dynamic Auscultation

DEFINITION

A cardiac murmur is defined as a relatively prolonged series of auditory vibrations of varying intensity, frequency, quality, configuration and duration.

CLASSIFICATION

There are three categories of murmurs:
1. Systolic,
2. Diastolic and
3. Continuous.

A diastolic murmur begins with or after the second heart sound and ends before the subsequent first heart sound. Diastolic murmurs are classified according to their time of onset as early diastolic, mid-diastolic or late diastolic.

1. **Early diastolic murmur** begins with the aortic or pulmonary component of the second heart sound, depending on its side of origin.
2. **Mid-diastolic murmur** begins at a clear interval after the second heart sound.
3. **Late diastolic or presystolic murmur** begins immediately before the first heart sound.

MECHANISM

Diastolic murmurs have two basic mechanisms of production. Diastolic filling murmurs or rumbles are due to forward flow across the atrioventricular valves, while diastolic regurgitant murmurs are due to retrograde flow across an incompetent semilunar valve.

EARLY DIASTOLIC MURMURS

An early diastolic murmur originating in the left side of the heart is exemplified by that heard in aortic regurgitation, while the pulmonary regurgitation murmur heard with pulmonary arterial hypertension represents one originating from the right side.

Aortic Regurgitation

Site: When the aortic regurgitation is valvular in origin, the murmur is best heard at the third and fourth left parasternal areas. If the murmur is best heard to the right of the sternum, it points to an aortic root etiology for the regurgitation; syphilis or Marfan's syndrome may be the cause.

Pitch and configuration: The pitch and character of the murmur is high frequency with decrescendo configuration. It is best appreciated with the patient sitting up and leaning forward and the diaphragm of the stethoscope firmly pressed against the chest wall. Since the pitch of the murmur approaches that of the respiratory sounds auscultation is carried out with the patient holding his breath after deep expiration. The murmur may be even louder in the high mid-left thorax, at the apex, or in the mid-axillary line rather than at the sternal edge. This has been called the *Cole-Cecil murmur*.

It begins with the aortic component of the second sound, i.e. as soon as the left ventricular pressure falls below the aortic incisura. The configuration of the murmur tends to reflect the volume and rate of regurgitant flow. Since the isovolumetric relaxation phase of the left ventricle is very rapid, a large gradient quickly develops between the aorta and the LV diastolic pressure, and the murmur builds up to a maximum intensity almost immediately after the aortic component. As diastole progresses the gradient between the two chambers falls slowly and the murmur follows the pressure drop in a decrescendo manner up to the first heart sound. The degree of aortic regurgitation is directly proportional to the pressure head driving the flow in a retrograde fashion.

Acute severe aortic regurgitation gives rise to a short diastolic murmur because the aortic diastolic pressure rapidly equilibrates with the steeply rising diastolic pressure in the unprepared non-dilated ventricle. The pitch of the murmur tends to be medium rather than high because the velocity of regurgitant flow is less rapid than in chronic severe aortic regurgitation.

Duration of the murmur: The murmur of very mild aortic regurgitation may be abbreviated and end by mid-diastole.

This is particularly true of the AR of systemic hypertension. As the volume of blood decreases in the aorta during diastole, the aortic ring becomes smaller and coupled with the decreasing aortic - LV diastolic gradient retrograde flow ceases and the murmur disappears.

The murmur of AR is also abbreviated if AR is acute. Acute regurgitation of blood into a ventricle that has not had time to adjust to a large volume load results in a marked elevation of LVEDP and equilibration of the aortic and LV diastolic pressures. With this retrograde flow ceases and the murmur disappears.

Dynamic auscultation: Maneuvers or pharmacological agents that increase or decrease the diastolic aortic-left ventricular pressure gradients will increase or decrease the murmur. Squatting, handgrip and the administration of vasopressors increase the intensity of the murmur by increasing the peripheral resistance. Inhalation of amyl nitrite decreases the intensity of the murmur. The murmur of mild aortic regurgitation often disappears during the latter stages of pregnancy due to the low peripheral resistance. The murmur is also decreased during the strain phase of the Valsalva maneuver due to the lower systolic pressure.

Severity of Aortic Regurgitation

The severity of the regurgitation correlates best with the duration rather than with the intensity of the murmur. In *mild AR* the murmur may be limited to early diastole and is typically high pitched and blowing. In *chronic AR* of a *moderate severity* the aortic diastolic pressure consistently and appreciably exceeds LV diastolic pressures, so the decrescendo murmur is subtle and the murmur is well heard throughout diastole. In chronic *severe aortic regurgitation* the decrescendo is more obvious paralleling the dramatic decline in aortic root diastolic pressure.

Musical Diastolic Murmur

The presence of a "cooing dove" or a musical diastolic murmur usually denotes a rupture or retroversion of a cusp. Such ruptures occur secondary to trauma, bacterial endocarditis and occasionally in the presence of arteriosclerotic involvement of the aortic valve. Retroversion and subsequent rupture of the aortic valve with a musical murmur is also a complication of syphilitic aortic regurgitation.

Sinus of Valsalva Aneurysms

A rupture into the left ventricle may cause an isolated murmur of aortic regurgitation. An unruptured aneurysm may also cause an isolated diastolic murmur of AR by interfering with cusp apposition.

Pulmonary Regurgitation

Early diastolic murmurs of the right side of the heart are represented by the Graham Steell murmur of pulmonary hypertensive pulmonary regurgitation. The murmur begins with a loud pulmonary component of the second heart sound; at the moment the right ventricular pressure drops below the pulmonary artery incisura. The high diastolic pressure generates high velocity regurgitant flow and results in a high frequency blowing murmur that may last throughout diastole. Due to the persistent and appreciable difference between pulmonary arterial and right ventricular pressures the amplitude of the murmur is usually relatively uniform throughout most of diastole

The frequency and the contour of the Graham Steell murmur is similar to that of aortic regurgitation because the hemodynamics are identical. These murmurs cannot be differentiated by either their quality or location on the chest wall. The differential is made from the company they keep. Careful investigation of the semilunar blowing murmur in the setting of mitral stenosis has shown that it is almost always due to aortic regurgitation even when significant pulmonary hypertension is present. More common causes of the Graham Steell murmur are primary pulmonary hypertension and Eisenmengers syndrome. When PA systolic pressures exceed 60 mmHg, dilatation of the annulus results in a regurgitant jet.

The murmur begins immediately after the P2 and is most prominent in the left parasternal region in the second to fourth intercostal spaces. It increases in intensity with inspiration and exhibits little change with amyl nitrite or vasopressors. It is diminished during the Valsalva strain and returns to baseline intensity immediately after the release of strain.

Table 1
Differentiation of aortic regurgitation and pulmonary regurgitation

Aortic regurgitation	Pulmonary regurgitation
P2 not loud	Loud P2
Normally split, Aortic component may be soft	Fused second heart sound
Peripheral signs of AR present	No peripheral signs of AR
Occurs immediately after A2	There is distinct gap after A2 and onset of murmur
No systolic murmur of TR	Systolic murmur of TR

Early diastolic murmurs are occasionally heard in end stage renal disease particularly when there is concurrent anemia, hypertension or fluid overload. These murmurs are usually pulmonary in origin. They are often transient in nature and are related to the fluid overload.

Dock's Murmur

Less common cause of EDM is a proximal LAD stenosis. It is not widely transmitted, usually best heard over the left second or third interspace, a little lateral to the left sternal border. This murmur is caused by turbulent flow across the coronary artery stenosis and its duration may be short or long. Following successful angioplasty or coronary artery bypass graft surgery, this murmur is abolished.

MID-DIASTOLIC MURMUR (MDM)

A mid-diastolic murmur begins at a clear interval after the second heart sound.

They originate from:
1. Stenosis of atrioventricular valve.
2. Increased flow across an unobstructed atrioventricular valve.
3. Pre-closure of AV valve.

Mitral Stenosis

Site: The murmur of mitral stenosis is best heard at the apex in the left lateral position with the bell of the stethoscope.

Intensity: It is related to the severity of the obstruction and to the flow across the valve. As a result there is poor correlation between the intensity of the murmur and the severity of the obstruction. High flow across a mild obstruction may produce a loud rumble, while low flow across a severely stenotic valve may produce a very soft murmur or may be silent.

The diastolic murmur of mitral stenosis may be masked by the presence of obesity, emphysema and a low cardiac output with a low flow rate across the mitral valve. The murmur may be sharply localized and thus missed. In so called *silent MS* there is usually marked right ventricular enlargement so that it occupies the cardiac apex. The LV is rotated posteriorly and the cardiac output is reduced so that the murmur is either not heard at all or can only be heard in the mid or posterior axillary line. The MS murmur also appears soft when present with a concomitant ASD, with severe PAH, with other valve obstructions like Aortic stenosis or Tricuspid stenosis, atrial fibrillation with a fast ventricular response or when there is an accompanying cardiomyopathy. A very dilated left atrium can lower the left atrial pressures even with severe MS and decrease the flow and therefore the loudness of the murmur.

Pitch and configuration: The murmur is described as a low-pitched rumbling murmur. The typical configuration of the murmur is a crescendo-decrescendo with a late crescendo up to M1. The murmur usually commences immediately after the mitral opening snap. When the murmur is soft it is limited to the apex but when louder it may radiate to the axilla or the lower left sternal area. The murmur persists as long as the left atrioventricular pressure gradient exceeds 3 mmHg.

The murmur is loudest in mid-diastole. As flow diminishes in late diastole the murmur tapers in intensity and may disappear. The presence or the absence of the murmur in late diastole is dependent on the magnitude of the LA-LV pressure gradient. In severe MS or with a rapid heart rate there is a continuous late diastolic gradient and a long diastolic murmur. If the mitral obstruction is only mild to moderate the LA may be decompressed and no gradient or murmur will be present in late diastole. The absence of a late diastolic component is most noticeable following long cycle lengths during atrial fibrillation or with slow heart rates in sinus rhythm.

Duration: The duration of the murmur is a guide to the severity of the disease. In mild MS the mid-diastolic murmur is brief but it resumes in presystole. In severe stenosis the murmur is holodiastolic with a presystolic accentuation in patients in sinus rhythm. In atrial fibrillation the duration of the mid-diastolic murmur is a useful sign of the degree of obstruction at the mitral orifice. A murmur that lasts up to the first heart sound even after long cycle lengths indicates that the stenosis is severe enough to generate a persistent gradient even at the end of long diastoles.

Dynamic auscultation: The diastolic murmur is reduced during inspiration and augmented during expiration. The diastolic rumble is reduced during the strain of Valsalva and in any condition in which the transmitral flow rate declines. Amyl nitrite, coughing accentuates a faint or equivocal murmur of MS.

Severity of Mitral Stenosis

Mild MS: There may either be a short mid-diastolic murmur or on occasion a presystolic crescendo murmur. If both murmurs are present there is usually a silent gap in mid to late diastole between the two audible murmur components.

Mild to moderate MS: Both the mid and late murmurs are readily heard but a distinct tapering or silence is observed after the mid-diastolic component.

Moderate to severe MS: With a persistent LA-LV gradient the diastolic rumble is truly pan-diastolic which starts from the opening snap lasting till the first heart sound, typically with an increase in intensity at end of diastole.

Table 2
Left-sided flow murmur

Mitral regurgitation
Ventricular septal defect
Patent ductus arteriosus
Aorto-pulmonary window
Rupture of a sinus of Valsalva aneurysm into the RV
Coarctation of the aorta and bicuspid aortic valve

Tricuspid Stenosis

Site: The murmur of tricuspid stenosis is usually heard in the xiphoid area just off the sternal edge.

Pitch and configuration: The murmur is usually softer, highre pitched and shorter in duration than the murmur of mitral stenosis. With sinus rhythm the murmur of TS tends to be mostly presystolic, however a mid-diastolic component was not uncommonly registered in severe cases, which is explained by a substantial gradient in mid-diastole in these cases.

With atrial fibrillation the characteristic murmur is mid-diastolic with a distinct decrescendo character especially in long diastolic intervals where the murmur may end long before the next cardiac cycle. In short diastolic cycles and with the presence of severe stenosis the murmur may occupy the whole of diastole. With inspiration there is a substantial increase in the intensity of the diastolic murmur of TS. A murmur of

Dynamic auscultation: The diastolic murmur is augmented by maneuvers that increase tricuspid flow like deep inspiration, the Mueller's maneuver, assumption of the right lateral decubitus position, leg raising, inhalation of amyl nitrite, squatting and isotonic exercise. It is reduced during expiration and during the strain of the Valsalva maneuver, and return to control level immediately (Within two or three beats) after Valsalva release.

Tricuspid regurgitation is almost invariably present with significant stenosis, with inspiration it was seen that the systolic murmur of TR was seen to appreciably diminish or not to change at all.

Table 3
Mid-diastolic murmur (MDM) at the mitral area

Atrial myxoma
Localized constrictive pericarditis of the atrioventricular ring
High flow across the atrioventricular valves–VSD or PDA
Rytands murmur
Carey Coombs murmur

Table 4
Mid-diastolic murmur (MDM) at the tricuspid area

Tricuspid regurgitation
Atrial septal defect
Anomalous pulmonary venous drainage

Rytand Murmur

Short mid-diastolic flow murmur occurs intermittently in complete heart block when atrial contraction coincides with the phase of rapid diastolic filling. These murmurs are believed to result from antegrade flow across A-V valves that are closing rapidly during filling of the recipient ventricle.

Carey Coombs Murmur

During an episode of rheumatic fever mitral valvulitis may cause a short mid-diastolic rumble. This rumble especially in children may be introduced by an S3 rather than an opening snap more so in the presence of anemia or fever. It is a soft early diastolic murmur that usually varies from day to day. It is high-pitched than the mid-diastolic rumble of mitral stenosis.

The soft apical mid-diastolic murmur is separated from the second heart sound by an appreciable gap representing the time interval between the aortic valve closure and the third heart sound. The murmur is best heard in the left lateral decubitus with the bell of the stethoscope. It is one of the few murmurs that is never accompanied by a thrill. The presence of the Carey Coomb murmur is seen to correlate with the later development of mitral stenosis on follow-up.

Flow Murmur

The mid-diastolic flow murmurs at the apex are usually heard when the shunt ratio is more than 2:1. The flow murmur differs from the MS murmur in that it usually starts with an S3 and there is no presystolic component. The mid-diastolic flow murmur across the tricuspid valve in an atrial septal defect does not increase with inspiration.

Pulmonary Regurgitation

A mid-diastolic murmur is a feature of pulmonary regurgitation with normal pulmonary arterial pressures. The murmur is best heard in the third and fourth left intercostal spaces in the parasternal area. It is a low pitched murmur, which commences when the pressures in the PA and the RV diverge, about 40 msec after the P2. It is crescendo-decrescendo in configuration ending well before the S1. It reaches a peak when the gradient between the pressures is maximal and ending after the equilibration of pressures. The murmur becomes louder after the inhalation of amyl nitrite or with inspiration. The diastolic pressure exerted upon the incompetent pulmonary valve is negligible at the inception of the pulmonary component of the second sound so the regurgitant flow is minimum. As the RV pressure dips below the diastolic pressure in the pulmonary trunk regurgitation accelerates and the murmur peaks. Late diastolic equilibration of RV and PA pressures eliminates regurgitant flow and abolishes the murmur prior to the next S1.

LATE DIASTOLIC OR PRESYSTOLIC MURMURS

A late diastolic murmur occurs immediately before the first heart sound. With few exceptions the late diastolic timing of the murmur coincides with the phase of ventricular filling that follows atrial systole and implies coordinated atrial contraction, generally sinus rhythm. Late diastolic or presystolic murmurs usually originate at the mitral or tricuspid valve because of the obstruction, but occasionally because of abnormal patterns of presystolic A-V flow.

Mitral Stenosis

The best-known presystolic murmur accompanies rheumatic mitral stenosis in sinus rhythm as AV flow is augmented in response to the increase in LA contraction. Presystolic accentuation of a mid-diastolic murmur is occasionally heard in mitral stenosis with atrial fibrillation especially during short cycle lengths. In patients with atrial fibrillation it results from the increased velocity of flow across a mitral valve orifice that begins to narrow after the onset of left ventricular contraction.

The presystolic murmur in mitral stenosis is crescendo in configuration increasing up to the first heart sound. Initially it was attributed only to an increase in flow across the valve but studies by Criley have suggested that it is actually due to high velocity antegrade flow through a progressively narrowing mitral orifice during the iso-volumetric contraction phase.

Tricuspid Stenosis

In sinus rhythm a late diastolic or presystolic murmur typically occurs in the absence of a perceptible mid-diastolic murmur. This is because the gradient is negligible until the powerful right atrial contraction. The presystolic murmur fades before the first heart sound. The murmur is augmented with inspiration. The presystolic murmur has a scratchy quality and occurs earlier than the one of mitral stenosis.

Complete Heart Block

Short presystolic crescendo-decrescendo murmurs are occasionally heard in complete heart block when atrial contraction falls in late diastole.

Austin Flint Murmur

This is a mid to late diastolic rumble heard over the apex in patients with severe aortic regurgitation which may occur with a normal mitral valve. In most cases of severe aortic regurgitation particularly when the regurgitation is acute the presystolic component of the murmur is lost. In this situation there is a marked increase in LVEDP and the reverse pressure gradient between the LV and the LA causes premature closure of the mitral valve.

Postulated *mechanisms* held responsible for the Austin Flint murmur include:

1. Late diastolic mitral regurgitation.
2. Isolated vibration of MV leaflets due to jet impinging on it.
3. Phonocardiographic studies have shown that the murmur is associated with rapid closing motion of the mitral valve leaflets during mid-diastole and presystole, the murmur being presumed to be due to antegrade flow across a closing orifice. This is the **most widely accepted mechanism, i.e. pre-closure of the mitral valve.**
4. The murmur has also been recorded in the absence of a rapid closure of the mitral valve where it was thought that incomplete valve opening rather than rapid closure being responsible for the increased mitral flow velocity.
5. One Echo-Doppler study has suggested that the murmur is due to the regurgitant jet being directed the mitral valve causing deformity and shuddering of the valve. This view is further supported by the presence of yellow plaques (jet lesions) on the septal surface of the anterior mitral leaflet.

The presence of the murmur indicates a large leak with a regurgitant fraction of greater than 50%. The pitch of the murmur is identical to that of the murmur of mitral stenosis and the murmur is typically preceded by an S3. It is best heard with the bell of the stethoscope.

Dynamic Auscultation

Infusion of vasopressors, isometric exercise, squatting and the application of bilateral blood pressure cuffs intensify the amplitude of the murmur. The murmur is diminished during the strain phase of Valsalva and inhalation of amyl nitrite.

Table 5
Difference between mitral MDM and Austin Flint murmur

	Mitral MDM murmur	*Austin flint murmur*
S1 loud	Present	No
P2 loud	Present	Rare
S3	Never	May be present
Opening snap	Present	No
Amyl nitrite	Murmur increases	Murmur decreases
Rhythm	May be AFib	Sinus rhythm
Peripheral signs of AR	None	Present
Apex beat	Tapping	Hyperdynamic

Right-Sided Austin Flint Murmur

This murmur has been reported with severe pulmonary regurgitation associated with pulmonary hypertension. It has not been noted with organic pulmonary regurgitation with a normal pulmonary arterial pressure.

Bioprosthetic Valve

A mid-diastolic murmur may be heard across a porcine valve due to the deflection of the blood flow through the valve towards the septum or the posterior ventricular wall rather than towards the apex. It is heard in about half the patients with a normally functioning porcine valve. Fluttering of the valves can be seen on Echocardiography.

CHAPTER 12

Continuous Murmurs

Oomen K George, Bobby John

CHAPTER OUTLINE

- Definition
- Mechanisms of Continuous Murmurs [Myer's Classification (1975)]
- Patent Ductus Arteriosus (Machinery murmur or Gibsons Murmur)
- Aortopulmonary Window
- Congenital Coronary Arterial Fistula
- Rupture of Sinus Valsalva Aneurysm
- Anomalous Origin of Left Coronary Artery from the Pulmonary Artery (Bland White Garland Syndrome)
- Congenital Pulmonary AV Fistula
- Acquired Arteriovenous Fistula
- Lutembacher Syndrome
- Murmurs Occurring in Constricted Arteries
- Continuous Murmur Arising from Collaterals between Systemic and Pulmonary Arteries
- Venous Hum
- Continuous Murmur with Cyanosis

DEFINITION

Murmurs that begin in systole and continue **without interruption through the second heart sound** into all or part of diastole are called continuous murmurs.

MECHANISMS OF CONTINUOUS MURMURS [Myer's Classification (1975)]

1. *Communication between a high-pressure and low-pressure zones.*
    - Patent ductus arteriosus
    - Aorto pulmonary window
    - Systemic to pulmonary shunts, e.g. Blalock Taussig, Waterston and Pott's shunt
    - Arteriovenous fistulas
        - Congenital
            - Intracranial
            - Hepatic
            - Lower and upper limbs.

- Acquired
    - Arteriovenous fistula of hemodialysis
    - Post traumatic
    - Surgery
    - Needle puncture
    - After cardiac catheterization.
- Rupture of sinus of valsalva into
    - Right atrium (RA)
    - Right ventricle (RV)
    - Left atrium (LA)
- Coronary cameral fistula
- Systemic to pulmonary arterial collaterals in cyanotic heart disease with diminished pulmonary blood flow
- Left to right atrial shunt MS with PFO or small ASD
- Cruveilhier Blumgarten Syndrome (Portal systemic shunt in cirrhosis)
- Anomalous left coronary from PA.

2. *Narrowing of an artery*
    - Coarctation of aorta
    - Renal artery stenosis
    - Peripheral pulmonary stenosis
    - Coronary stenosis
    - TAPVC infradiaphragmatic/intracardiac
    - Aortoarteritis (Takayasu's disease).

3. *Increased velocity of flow with turbulence*
    - The cervical venous hum
    - Over the skull in children with anemia
    - TAPVC—Supracardiac
    - Bronchial artery dilatation associated with pulmonary atresia, pulmonary hypertension or coarctation of aorta.

4. *Increased blood flow to an organ*
    - Thyrotoxicosis
    - Hypernephroma
    - Hepatoma
    - Mammary souffle
    - Hemangioma.

PATENT DUCTUS ARTERIOSUS (MACHINERY MURMUR OR GIBSONS MURMUR)

The murmur of uncomplicated patent ductus arteriosus (PDA) rises to a peak in latter systole, continues without interruption through the second heart sound, which it envelops and then decreases in intensity during diastole.

High velocity flow through a small restrictive PDA causes a soft high frequency murmur. Larger restrictive PDAs produce a noisy machinery murmur accentuated in latter systole and punctuated with Eddy Sounds (multiple clicks) in latter systole. There is early collision of streams from the ductus and pulmonary artery. The murmur is best heard in the first or second left intercostal space or beneath the left clavicle. The term rough and thrilling applies to this type of PDA murmur. The PDA murmur is increased by Methoxamine and attenuated by Amyl Nitrite. With the development of pulmonary hypertension in large RDA, the diastolic component starts to disappear and only the systokic component may remain. Right to left shunt across a PDA does not produce a murmur.

AORTOPULMONARY WINDOW

Only 20% of aortopulmonary (AP) windows are associated with continuous murmurs because most of the AP windows are nonrestrictive and pulmonary pressures are elevated which abolishes the diastolic component. When continuous murmur is present, it tends to be short. Patients with restrictive AP windows have a long continuous murmur, identical to PDA murmur classically heard in the third left intercostal space, but can be one space above or below which causes confusion with a PDA or VSD murmur.

CONGENITAL CORONARY ARTERIAL FISTULA

This condition should always be suspected when an acyanotic individual presents with a continuous murmur maximal at an atypical precordial site. About 50% of these fistulae involve the right coronary artery, and 45% left coronary artery. Site of the murmur depends on the chamber, which receives the flow. About 90% drain into the right side of the heart.

Usually, the continuous murmurs of coronary artery fistula are soft (Grade III or less with high frequency), as they carry small shunt through a narrow pathway. Exceptionally, they produce coarse rough and machinery murmurs when the fistula is large. The murmur is louder either in systole or diastole. They sometimes resemble a PDA murmur by configuration, however, the site of the murmur helps in differentiation. The Valsalva manoeuvre increases the right-sided pressures and softens the murmur.

General Principles

When the fistula drains into the **RA, coronary sinus or left atrium,** the pressure gradient between aortic root and receiving chamber are larger during systole than during diastole. The volume and rate of flow through the fistula tend to parallel the gradients, so that the murmur is likely to be ***louder in systole***.

When the fistula communicates with **pulmonary trunk**, flow is also greater in systole. But the difference is less marked.

Table 1
Location of murmur according to the chamber, which receives the flow

Chamber	Site of murmur
Right Ventricle	Mid to lower left sternal border or over the lower sternum
RV Outflow Tract	Mid to upper left sternal edge
Right Atrium	Mid to lower right sternal edge & over the lower sternum
Pulmonary Trunk	Left 2nd or 3rd Intercostal space along the sternal border
Left Atrium	Upper to mid left sternal border may radiate up to anterior axillary line

The accompanying murmur can be *louder in systole.* But may increase around the second heart sound as in PDA.

When the **RV** receives the fistulous coronary artery, the flow patterns are more complex. Contraction of the ventricle variably compresses the fistulous coronary artery as it passes through the ventricular wall to its drainage site. Marked compression reduces systolic flow and causes the murmur to *soften in systole.* However, if the lumen of fistula is only narrowly compressed, the systolic gradient across its constricted intramural portion increases. The continuous murmur is then *louder in systole.*

RUPTURE OF SINUS VALSALVA ANEURYSM

Sudden appearance of superficial, loud sawing continuous murmur in a previously healthy individual which does not peak around second heart sound, the systolic or the diastolic component being louder suggest the presence of rupture of sinus of valsalva (RSOV) to right side of the heart. The diastolic component can be made louder by increasing aortic systolic pressure during isometric handgrip or valsalva release. The site of the murmur depends on whether the rupture is into RA, RV or RVOT.

RSOV into RA

When the RA receives the perforation, the continuous murmur is maximal adjacent to the right or left sternal border or over the lower sternum.

RSOV into RV

When the rupture enters the *body of RV*, the murmur is heard best at the mid to lower left sternal border. Rupture into RV *near the tricuspid orifice* may be associated with a continuous murmur at the right sternal edge. Perforation into *outflow tract* results in a murmur site higher along the left sternal edge. The systolic component of the continuous murmur tends to be louder at higher thoracic levels and the diastolic component tends to be louder at lower levels.

ANOMALOUS ORIGIN OF LEFT CORONARY ARTERY FROM THE PULMONARY ARTERY (BLAND WHITE GARLAND SYNDROME)

The continuous murmur is variably located to the left or right of sternum at the base of the heart or somewhat lower, softer in systole and louder in diastole. The murmur is generated by collateral flow between RCA and LCA, which decreases due to compression, by increased transmural pressure during LV systole. Some patients have associated PDA, MR or LVF, which elevates the pulmonary arterial pressure and abolishes the diastolic component of this continuous murmur.

ECG would show deep Q waves in lead I, aVL and V4 to V6. LVH is also an important electrocardiographic finding in patients with ALCAPA.

CONGENITAL PULMONARY AV FISTULA

This condition can give rise to a continuous murmur with a louder systolic component over the lower lobes and middle lobe of the right lung. The murmur increases on inspiration, standing and Muller manoeuvre. It decreases during Valsalva manoeuvre.

ACQUIRED ARTERIOVENOUS FISTULA

Acquired arteriovenous fistula can occur as a result of trauma or can be surgically created for hemodialysis. A loud continuous murmur with systolic accentuation is usually present with maximum intensity at or around the site of fistula. Manual compression of the fistula can lead to reflex bradycardia.

LUTEMBACHER SYNDROME

When tight mitral stenosis coexists with a restrictive interatrial communication, the left to right shunt is continuous because an appreciable pressure difference exists across the interatrial communication throughout the cardiac cycle. The murmur is heard at the lower right sternal edge because the murmur is generated with the cavity of the right atrium. The continuous murmur may increase with inspiration, a response ascribed to a late inspiratory rise in left atrial pressure.

MURMURS OCCURRING IN CONSTRICTED ARTERIES

For a constricted arterial segment to produce a continuous murmur there should be critical narrowing with inadequate collaterals which will lead to a systolic and diastolic gradient across the narrowing. An atherosclerotic carotid artery or femoral artery occasionally produces a continuous murmur.

Pulmonary artery branch stenosis can produce a continuous murmur when there is higher pressure proximal to the stenosis with inadequate collateral flow. The murmur is heard outside the cardiac dullness. Narrowing of the origin pulmonary artery in Truncus arteriosus can produce a continuous murmur.

Mammary soufflé: Occurs in 10–15% of pregnant women in late pregnancy and early post partum. It is louder in systole and maximal over either lactating breast between the second and sixth left intercostal space.

CONTINUOUS MURMUR ARISING FROM COLLATERALS BETWEEN SYSTEMIC AND PULMONARY ARTERIES

1. ***TOF with pulmonary atresia:*** Direct and indirect systemic arterial collaterals produce continuous murmurs in 80% of cases. The intensity varies from soft to readily detectable murmur. Usual sites are beneath the clavicle, back, right or left side of chest or equally on both sides.
2. ***Multiple peripheral pulmonary artery stenosis:*** Bronchial collateral enlarge and can produce continuous murmurs.
3. ***Truncus arteriosus (Type III):*** Bronchial collaterals to the side of hypoplastic pulmonary arteries rarely cause a continuous murmur.
4. In advanced bronchiectasis and sequestrated lung bronchopulmonary collaterals can lead to a continuous murmur.
5. Intercostal collaterals may cause a continuous murmur in coarctation of aorta. Collaterals between the ascending and descending aorta can cause continuous murmur in aortic arch interruption.

VENOUS HUM

This murmur described by Potain in 1867 is the most common continuous murmur. It is universal in young children and frequent in healthy young adults, especially in pregnancy. Thyrotoxicosis and anemia reinforce a venous hum. It is rough and noisy occasionally associated with a high-pitched whine. The murmur is typically louder in diastole, best heard in the right supraclavicular fossa lateral to sternocleidomastoid. The murmur of venous hum is increased by upright position, deep inspiration and during diastole. If venous hum is audible in supine position suspect a hyperdynamic circulatory state.

Two Mechanisms Proposed for Venous Hum

Anterior angulation of the internal jugular vein at the transverse process of atlas.

Turbulance caused by confluence of flow through the IJV and subclavian vein as they pour into the superior vena cava.

Total Anomalous Pulmonary Venous Connection

Here the murmur has the quality of a soft venous hum, but it is not louder in diastole. Site—upper left sternal border. Mild to moderate obstruction to the venous confluence in presence of increased flow increases this murmur.

Hepatic Venous Hum

This is heard over the liver and disappears with pressure over the epigastrium.

CONTINUOUS MURMUR WITH CYANOSIS

- TOF with Pulmonary Atresia.
- Total anomalous pulmonary venous connection with obstructed vertical vein
- Congenital pulmonary AV fistula
- Severe peripheral pulmonary stenosis
- Truncus arteriosus with narrow origin of pulmonary arteries/Bronchial collaterals.
- Pulmonary atresia with intact ventricular septum with anomalous origin of LCA from pulmonary trunk.

CHAPTER 13

Rheumatic Fever

Jacob Jose

CHAPTER OUTLINE

- Group a beta hemolytic streptococci (GABHS)
- Criteria for diagnosis
- Arthritis
- Carditis
- Chorea
- Preceding streptococcal infection within last 45 days Mandatory Criteria
- Treatment

Acute rheumatic fever (RF) is a major health problem in developing countries like India despite the fact that there has been a dramatic decline in USA and Europe. RF is a sequel to Streptococcal infection.

GROUP A BETA HEMOLYTIC STREPTOCOCCI - GABHS

- RF is caused GABHS infection of the upper respiratory tract.
- Certain M types have been thought to be rheumatogenic (1, 3, 5, 6, 14, 18, 19, 27 and 29).
- The attack rate of Rheumatic fever is **3% in epidemics but in populations it is around 0.3%.**
- A strong relationship has been found with a B-cell antigen designated 883; this is found in patients with rheumatic fever suggesting that there could be a genetic predisposition. Some HLA antigens such as HLA – DR 7 and HLA – DR 4 have been associated with susceptibility and HLA – DR 5,6,51 and 52 have been associated with protection.
- Familial clustering of cases of chorea have been noted particularly for chorea in twins.

Prevalence of Rheumatic Heart Disease in India

In order to understand the prevalence of rheumatic heart disease, we can get data either from school surveys or hospital admissions. **Table 1** gives the school survey data regarding the prevalence of rheumatic heart disease in India. As shown in the table, **the prevalence varies from 0.68 to 4.54 per thousand school children.**

Table 1
School survey data of rheumatic heart disease from India

Author	Place	Year	Age	Population studied	Prevalence/1000
ICMR [1]	Vellore	1982–1990	5–15	13,509	2.9
Padmavati [2]	Delhi (urban)	1984–1994	5–10	40,000	3.9
Grover [3]	Raipurrani	1988–1991	5–15	31,200	2.1
Avasthi [4]	Ludhiana	1987	6–16	6,005	1.3
Patel [5]	Anand	1986	8–18	11,346	2.03
Lalchandani [6]	Kanpur	2000	7–15	3,963	4.54
Jacob Jose [7]	Vellore	2003	5–18	2,29,829	0.68
Anita Saxena [8]	Delhi	2011	5–15	6,270	0.8

Age of RF

The most common five percent age at presentation is between 5 to 15 years of age. 5% of cases can occur in less than 5 years. **The earliest age at which RF is reported** is 1.9 years.[9] It is usually stated that RF does not occur after the age of 40 years but one case has been reported at the age of 90 years.[10]

CRITERIA FOR DIAGNOSIS

For the diagnosis of acute rheumatic fever, we have been following the Jones criteria, since 1944. However, there are many patients who do not fulfill the Jone's criteria and presently, a new dimension has been added with advent of echocardiography. Echocardiogram is able to identify valve lesions that are not present clinically – sub-clinical carditis. The current guidelines for diagnosis of RF was revised and published in the year 2015 **(Tables 2 to 4)**.[11]

Table 2
2015 Revised Jones criteria for low risk population

Major manifestations	Minor manifestations
Carditis: Clinical or subclinical	
Arthritis: Polyarthritis only	Polyarthragia
Chorea	Fever 38.5°C
Subcutaneous nodules	ESR >60 or CRP >3
Erythema marginatum	Prolonged PR interval

RF incidence is <2 per 1,00,000 in school going age and RHD prevalence is 1 or less per 1000 population per year

Table 3
2015 Revised Jones criteria for moderate or high-risk population

Major manifestations	Minor manifestations
Carditis: Clinical or subclinical	
Arthritis: Mono or Polyarthritis or polyarthralgia	Monoarthralgia
Chorea	Fever 38°
Subcutaneous nodules	ESR > 30 mm/h or CRP > 3
Erythema marginatum	Prolonged PR interval

Low risk is defined as RF incidence is < 2 per 100,000 in school going age and RHD prevalence is 1 or less per 1000 population per year

Table 4
Revised Jones criteria for diagnosis of RF

Preceding GAS infection plus	
First episode	2 major or 1 major and 2 minor
Recurrent without RHD	2 major or 1 major + 2 minor or 3 minor

In the above criteria there are 5 major, 4 minor and we need a supporting evidence of preceding group A streptococcal infection. **This supporting evidence** can be a positive throat culture or elevated or rising streptococcal antibody titer.

Exceptions to Jones Criteria

1. Chorea.
2. Indolent carditis.
3. Recurrent rheumatic fever.
4. Post-streptoccocal arthritis.

ARTHRITIS

1. Occurs in 70% of cases.
2. Asymmetrical and **migratory** in nature
3. Large joint arthritis (Knees, ankles, elbows and wrist are involved).
4. Pain, swelling, heat, and redness are noted. **Pain is disproportionately greater than effusion**.
5. Lasts for 2–3 weeks.
6. Rapid response to salicylates within 48 hours.
7. *No residual deformity* If untreated the inflammatory findings last from **1 to 5 days in each joint**, reach the highest intensity in the first 2 days, with the entire process subsiding over 2 to 4 weeks. Involvement of only one joint is observed if anti-inflammatory therapy is given before the migratory pattern is established.

8. PSRA has short latent period, small joints also involved, and persistence of mono or polyarthritis for several months.
9. In the 2015 guidelines, polyarthralgia has been added as a major criteria and monoarthralgia is added as a minor criterion.

Other causes for migratory polyarthritis (NEJM March 17, 1994; 769)
   1. Rheumatic fever
   2. Gonococcemia
   3. Meningococcemia
   4. Viral arthritis
   5. SLE
   6. Acute leukemia
   7. Whipples disease.

Jaccoud's Arthritis

This is a permanent deformity of small joints, secondary to rheumatic fever, which is very rare. This is also described in SLE and other connective tissue diseases. The deformity is due to soft tissue abnormalities such as laxity of ligaments, fibrosis of the capsule and muscular imbalance and not due to destruction of joints.

CARDITIS

Carditis occurs in 50% of patients with acute rheumatic fever. In Indian scenario the incidence of carditis is higher than the western data (range 70-86%). Since carditis includes some or one of the following, the features are given in increasing order of severity.
1. Tachycardia (out of proportion to the degree of fever) is common; its absence makes the diagnosis of myocarditis unlikely.
2. A heart murmur of valvulitis [caused by mitral regurgitation (MR) and/or aortic regurgitation (AR)] is almost always present; **without the murmurs of MR and/or AR, carditis should not be diagnosed.**
   Mechanism of MR: Chordal elongation or due to annular dilatation of mitral valve.
3. Pericarditis (friction rub, pericardial effusion, chest pain, and ECG changes) may be present.
4. Cardiomegaly on chest X-ray films is indicative of pericarditis, pancarditis, or congestive heart failure (CHF).
5. Signs of congestive heart failure (gallop rhythm, distant heart sounds, cardiomegaly) are indications of severe carditis.

6. **Myocarditis is unlikely due to the following reasons in RF**.[12] Absence of myocarditis has been documented by: (i) No increase in markers of myocardial damage –CK MB, Troponin I & T and myoglobin. (ii) Normal LV systolic function and myocardial contractility by echocardiographic studies. (iii) Radionuclide studies using technetium pyrophosphate scanning and indium labelled anticardiac myocin Fab (FAB) do not indicate presence of myocardial damage. (iv) Myocardial biopsy studies have not been able to identify the presence of myocarditis. (v) Normalization of heart size and disappearance of congestive failure following surgical mitral and/or aortic valve replacement in patients deteriorating in spite of aggressive medical management. (vi) Histopathology of the LV myocardium shows absence of myocardial or intermyocardial connective tissue damage. (vii) Immunopathology of Aschoff nodule (AN), the diagnostic marker of rheumatic pathology, being derived from mesenchymal cells, and absence of actin, myosin and desmin (of myocardial origin) in the AN nodule indicating that AN is not of myocardial origin. **Hence, congestive cardiac failure in acute RF is due to an acute volume overload from mitral and/or aortic regurgitation but not due to myocarditis** *per se.*

Valve Involvement in Acute Rheumatic Fever

- Mitral – 70–75%
- Mitral and Aortic – 20–25%
- Aortic – Isolated 5%.

Valve Combinations in Indian Data for Chronic RHD (IHJ 2014: 320- 326)

- MS + MR: 46%
- MS + AR: 26%
- MR + AR: 23%
- MS+ AS: 2.4%
- MR + AS: 0.3%

Carditis—Role of Echo

It is difficult to clinically diagnose mild carditis. Echocardiogram is a valuable tool for the diagnosis of a valvular lesion. Echo is capable of evaluating the presence and degree of mitral and aortic regurgitation. The first report regarding the role of echo was by Steinfield in the year 1986. He found that Doppler showed mitral regurgitation even when there was clinically no murmur.[13] Echo Doppler is extremely useful in the diagnosis of carditis by identifying valvular disease even in patients without clinical evidence of carditis. The increasing role of Echo in the criteria formation is highlighted in Table 5. Criteria that are used to identify the pathological regurgitations and morphological criteria for the same are given in Tables 6 and 7. Dr Vijayalakshmi from Jayadeva Institute has suggested another useful criteria for Echo and this is given in Table 8.

Table 5
Role of echo in the diagnosis of RF

Year	Guidelines	Echo is recommended
1992	Jones criteria updated	No
2001	WHO guidelines	Yes
2008	Indian Working Group	Yes
2008	New Zealand	Yes
2012	Australian	Yes
2015	Revised Jones criteria	Yes

Table 6
Echo Doppler criteria in rheumatic valvulitis

Valve	Doppler Findings (all 4 criteria to be met)
Mitral valve	Seen in 2 views 2 cm in length Peak velocity >3 m/sec Pan systolic in at least 1 envelope
Aortic valve	Seen in 2 views 1 cm in length or more Peak velocity > 3 m/sec Pans diastolic in at least 1 envelope

Table 7
Morphological findings in echo criteria for valvulitis

Acute mitral valve changes	• Annular dilation • Chordal elongation • Chordal rupture • Anterior leaflet prolapse • Beading or nodularity of leaflets
Chronic mitral valve changes	• Leaflet thickening • Chordal thickening • Restricted leaflet motion • Calcification
Aortic valve changes in either acute or chronic	• Irregular or focal leaflet thickening • Cooptation defect • Restricted leaflet motion • Leaflet prolapse

Table 8
Echo criteria for the diagnosis of carditis[14]

	Echo feature	Score
1	Thickness of mitral and aortic leaflets greater than 4 mm	2
2	Increased echogenicity of submitral structures	2
3	Rheumatic nodules, giving beaded appearance	2
4	Prolapse of mitral, aortic or tricuspid valves	2
5	Mitral, aortic or tricuspid regurgitation	2
6	Reduced mobility of leaflets	2
7	Chordal tear	2
8	Pericardial effusion	
	Total Score	16

Vijaya's -Score of more than 6 out of 16 is required)

CHOREA

Also called as **Sydenham's chorea, or St Vitus dance** is the **third** most common major manifestation. It occurs in **15%** of patients in recent outbreaks; however, the overall figure may be around 5% or less. The period of latency between the GABHS infection and the onset of chorea is around **3 months.**

Chorea can occur in two circumstances:
1. As an isolated manifestation of rheumatic fever and frequently recurs following a new bout of streptococcal pharyngitis. This is called as **Pure chorea.**
2. It may occur as a part of otherwise active Rheumatic fever with manifestations such as joint pains, etc.

After puberty, chorea is almost entirely seen only in women. It may last for a few weeks to few months. It seems to be due to immune mediated reaction to autoantibodies of the basal ganglia. Severe chorea responds to treatment with intravenous IgG.

The clinical findings include involuntary and purposeless movements with muscle in coordination of the extremities and labile mood.

Signs

1. Hyperextension of the fingers, **spooning** when the arms are extended
2. **Pronation** of hands when arms are raised vertically.
3. **Milkmaid's** grip—Irregular contraction of the hand muscles when the patient presses the hand of the examiner.
4. **Wormian tongue**—Gross fasciculations of the tongue when extended.
5. Clumsiness in fine movements such as buttoning of the shirt.

Duration

Usually self-limited and last for 2 – 4 weeks; can last for a few months to 2 years.

Sequelae

1. Studies suggest that many patients with chorea may eventually have obsessive-compulsive behavior. No residual neurological deficit is seen in most patients.
2. When chorea is associated with other signs of RF, the incidence of valve damage is comparable to that caused by other patients without chorea.
3. When chorea is an isolated event – pure chorea, the valve damage is less frequent and mitral stenosis is the late manifestation.

PRECEDING STREPTOCOCCAL INFECTION WITHIN LAST 45 DAYS—MANDATORY CRITERIA

- Positive **throat culture** is **less reliable** than streptococcal antibody test because they do not differentiate between recent throat infection and chronic pharyngeal carrier.
- **Streptococcal antibody tests** are the most reliable laboratory evidence for receiving streptococcal infection. The onset of clinical manifestations of acute rheumatic fever coincides with the peak of streptococcal antibody response. **Antistreptolysin O (ASO) titer** is the one that is used routinely. It is elevated in 80% of patients with acute rheumatic fever and in 20% of normal individuals. Only 67% of patients with isolated chorea have an elevated ASO titer. **ASO titer of at least 333 Todd units in children and 250 Todd units in adults are considered in elevated. It is better to use local data if available. Table 9 is the cutoff value from the Australian guidelines.**
- If the clinical suspicion is high but the ASO titer is low, this does not exclude the diagnosis of acute rheumatic fever. You must do one more test such as antideoxyribonuclease

Table 9

ULN for serum streptococcal antibody titers in children and adults

Age group	ULN (U/ml) Todds units	
Years	ASO tit	Anti-DNase B tit
1–4	170	366
5–14	276	499
15–24	238	473
25–34	177	390
≥35	127	265

B test (ADNB) or repeat the ASO titer after a week. A rising titer of ASO can be taken as evidence for RF. Streptozyme test is relatively simple agglutination test but it is less standardized and less reproducible than the other antibody test. It **should not be used** as a definitive test.

Clinical Course

1. Only carditis can cause permanent cardiac damage. Signs of mild carditis disappear rapidly in weeks, but those of severe carditis may last for 2 to 6 months.
2. Arthritis subsides within a few days to several weeks, even without treatment, and does not cause permanent damage.
3. Chorea gradually subsides in 6 to 7 months or longer and usually does not cause permanent neurological sequelae.

TREATMENT

1. Eradication of streptococci.
2. Anti-inflammatory drugs: Salicylates or Steroids for symptomatic relief.
3. Bed rest.
4. Secondary prophylaxis.

Eradication of streptococci: AHA statement—Circulation March 2009[15]

1. Injection **Benzathine Penicillin G:** 0.6 million units if the weight is < 27 kg or 1.2 million units if the weight is > 27 kg—single dose.
2. Oral Penicillin V 250 mg thrice daily 10 days.
3. Amoxycillin 50 mg/kg daily oral for 10 days **once daily.**
4. **In patients allergic to penicillin** Cephalexin group for 10 days OR Azithromycin for 5 days once daily 12 mg/kg OR Clarithromycin for 5 days given twice daily – 15 mg/kg/day OR Clindamycin thrice daily for 10 days – 20 mg/kg/day
   - With **allergic to penicillin – not type 1, can be given Cephalosporin or clindamycin. The macrolides such as azithromycin are deemphasized** because there is increasing resistance of GAS to this group of antibiotics and they are not as well tolerated, often provoking gastrointestinal symptoms.
   - For those with **severe type 1 allergy to penicillin, clindamycin should be the first choice.**

The following drugs are not acceptable:
1. Sulfonamides
2. Trimethoprim
3. Tetracyclines
4. Fluroquinolones

2. Anti-inflammatory drugs

Salicylates or Steroids must not be started until a definitive diagnosis is made. Early therapy with these drugs may interfere with definitive diagnosis of acute rheumatic fever (Flowchart 1). The role of steroids is controversial since we do not have any studies that have been done in the last 40 years with steroids. However, it is a common practice to use steroids with moderate to severe carditis.

- Severe carditis: Prednisolone 2 mg/kg/day
- Moderate carditis: Prednisolone 1–2 mg/kg/day
- Mild carditis: Aspirin 75–100 mg/kg/day in 4 divided doses.
- Polyarthritis: Aspirin 75–100 mg/kg/day in 4 divided doses or Naproxen 10–20 mg/kg/day.

3. Bed rest of varying duration is recommended. The duration depends on the severity of the clinical manifestation. ESR is a helpful guide to the rheumatic activity and therefore the duration of restriction of activities. Tables 10 and 11 will give you a general guidelines for bed rest/restricted ambulation period.

4. Secondary prevention of rheumatic fever: Tables 12 and 13 give the dose and the duration for secondary prophylaxis.

Table 10
Duration of anti-inflammatory agents

Clinical manifestation	Prednisolone	Aspirin
Arthritis alone	0	1–2 weeks
Mild carditis	0	3–4 weeks
Moderate carditis	0	6–8 weeks
Severe carditis	2–6 weeks*	6 weeks to 4 months

*For severe carditis, prednisolone should be tapered and Aspirin be started during the final week. To prevent rebound phenomenon. This can appear during the withdrawal of steroids. It may be clinical with exacerbation of symptoms and signs of ARF or biochemical with elevation of laboratory inflammatory markers such as ESR or CRP.

Table 11
General guidelines of restricted activities in acute rheumatic fever

Clinical feature	Duration of bed rest/limited ambulation
Arthritis alone	Only 2 weeks
Mild carditis	3-4 weeks
Moderate carditis (definite but mild cardiomegaly)	4-6 weeks
Severe carditis (marked cardiomegaly, cardiac failure, pericardial effusion)	Bed rest as long as patient has heart failure and indoor ambulation for a period of 2-3 months

Table 12
Drugs used in secondary prophylaxis

Drug	Dose	Route
1. Benzathine Penicillin G	1.2 million units every 3-4 weeks	IM
2. Penicillin V	250 mg twice daily	PO
3. Sulfadiazine	0.5 gm once daily for patients < 27 kg OR 1.0 gm once daily for patients > 27kg	PO
4. Allergic to penicillin and sulfadiazine	Erythromycin 250 mg twice daily	PO

Table 13
Duration of secondary prophylaxis

	ACC/AHA 2014	WHO Tech report 923
RF with carditis and residual heart disease	At least 10 years or until 40 years of age	Lifelong
RF with carditis with no residual heart disease	10 years or up to 21 years of age whichever is longer	10 years or up to 25 years whichever is longer
RF without carditis	5 years or up to 21 years of age whichever is longer	5 years or up to 18 years of age whichever is longer

3 weekly regimen of Benzathine Penicillin is **justified and recommended** for countries like India where the incidence of RF is high.

Rheumatic Fever Recurrence Rates using Drugs

- 3 weekly Benzathine Penicillin   0.25/100 person years
- 4 weekly Benzathine Penicillin   1.29/100 person years
- Sulfonamides   2.8/100 person years
- Oral Penicillin   5.5/100 person years

Since risk of recurrence is higher with oral penicillin, it is usually given for individuals who have reached young adulthood and remained free of rheumatic attacks for at least 5 years.

Treatment of Chorea

1. Phenobarbitol: 15–30 mg every 6th hourly.
2. Haloperidol: 2 mg every 8th hourly or as needed.
3. Sodium Valproate: 20 mg/kg/day in divided doses.

Flowchart Treatment for Rheumatic fever

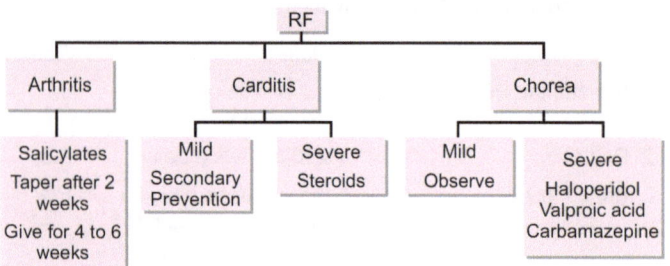

CONCLUSION

Acute rheumatic fever and rheumatic heart disease still forms a major health problem in countries like India. Early diagnosis and proper treatment of the disorder will prevent the marked disability left behind by this disease. We as clinicians should take an active role for prevention of this disease from India.

REFERENCES

1. Pilot study on the feasibility of utilizing the existing school health services in Delhi for the control of RF/RHD. ICMR final report, 1990.
2. Padmavati S. Present status of rheumatic fever and rheumatic heart disease in India. Indian Heart J. 1995; 47:395-8.
3. Grover A, Dhawan A, Iyengar SD, Anand IS, Wahi PL, Ganguly NK. Epidemiology of rheumatic fever and rheumatic heart disease in a rural community in northern India. Bull World Health Organ. 1993;71:59-66.
4. Avasthi G, Singh D, Singh C, Aggarwal SP, Bidwai PS, Avasthi R. Prevalence survey of rheumatic fever (RF) and rheumatic heart disease (RHD) in urban and rural school children in Ludhiana. Indian Heart J. 1987;39:26-8.
5. Patel DC, Pael NI, Patel JD, Patel SD. Rheumatic fever and rheumatic heart disease in school children of Anand. J Assoc Physicians India. 1986;34:837-9.
6. Lalchandani A, Kumar HRP, Alam SM. Prevalence of rheumatic fever and rheumatic heart disease in rural and urban school children of district Kanpur [Abstr]. Indian Heart. 2000;52:672.
7. Jose, et al. Declining prevalence of rheumatic heart disease in rural school children in India:2001-2002. IHJ. 2003;158-60.
8. Saxena A, et al. RHEUMATIC study. Heart. 2011;97:2018-22.
9. Lloyd Y Tani, et al. Rheumatic fever in children younger than 5 years. Pediatrics. 2003;112:1065-8.
10. Kasitanon, et al. Acute rheumatic fever in adults. Rheumatol Int. 2009;29:1041-5.
11. AHA scientific statement – Revision of the Jones criteria. Circulation. 2015;131:1806-18.

12. Kumar K, Tandon. Rheumatic fever &rheumatic heart disease: the last 50 years. Indian Journal of Medical Research, 2013;137:643-58.
13. Steinfield, Ritter S, Rapport H, Martinez E-Silent Rheumatic Mitral regurgitation unmasked by Doppler studies. Abstract – Circulation. 1986;74:11:385.
14. Vijyalakshmi et al. The efficacy of Echo criterions for the diagnosis of acute rheumatic fever. Cardiology Young. 2008;18:586-92.
15. Gerber et al. AHA scientific statement. Circulation. 2009;119: 1541-51.

CHAPTER 14

Aortic Stenosis

Jacob Jose

CHAPTER OUTLINE

- Hemodynamics
- Etiology of Valvar AS
- History
- Physical Findings
- Chest X-Ray
- ECG
- Echo Assessment of AS
- Natural History
- Surgery
- Statins and Aortic Stenosis Progression
- Low Flow Low Gradient AS
- Aortic Stenosis with Regurgitation
- Transcatheter Aortic Valve Replacement—TAVI

The normal aortic valve has **three layers** anatomically. The layer facing the left ventricle is called as **Ventricularis.** This is made up of elastin fibers aligned in a radial direction, perpendicular to the leaflet margin. The layer facing the aortic side is called as **fibrosa**; in this, the fibers are arranged parallel to the leaflet margin. The third layer is called **spongiosa**, it is seen between the fibrosa and ventricularis at the base of the leaflet. This layer is made up of fibroblasts, mesenchymal cells and is rich in mucopolysaccharides.

■ HEMODYNAMICS

In aortic stenosis (AS), there is obstruction to left ventricular outflow. The valve area is reduced from the normal of 2.6–3.4 sq cm. As a result of the valve narrowing, there is a gradient across the valve and **compensatory hypertrophy** of the LV. The hemodynamic changes in AS are summarized below:
- LV Systolic pressure is increased
- LV Ejection time is increased
- LV End diastolic pressure is increased
- Gradient across the valve
- Aortic mean pressure is decreased.

Table 1 shows the grading of aortic stenosis by the ESC Echo guidelines and Table 2 shows the relationship between the aortic valve area and mean gradient. **As the severity of aortic stenosis increases there is quadrupling of the mean gradient.**

Table 1
Grading of AS according to European Society of Echo guidelines 2009[1]

	Aortic sclerosis	Mild	Moderate	Severe
Jet Velocity m/sec	<2.5	2.6–2.9	3–4	>4
Mean gradient mmHg		<20	20–40	>40
Valve area sq cm		>1.5	1–1.5	<1

Table 2
Mean gradient and AVA in AS with constant cardiac output 5 liter/minute

Aortic valve area sq cm	Mean gradient mm Hg
1.5	14
1.0	21
0.7	42
0.5	82

ETIOLOGY OF VALVAR AS

- Congenital
- Rheumatic
- Calcific (degenerative) is now the most common cause of severe AS
- Rarely (Homozygous hyperlipidemia, rheumatoid, ochrnosis).

Congenital AS: The valve may be unicuspid, bicuspid or tricuspid. Unicuspid valves produce severe AS in infancy. Tricuspid valves develop AS over a period of time and they manifest only at 30 years of age or more.

Bicuspid AV is one of the commonest congenital lesions occurring **in 2% of live births**. However in a study done in 1,075 neonates **by Echo the prevalence was 4.6 per 1,000 live births**. In 80% of cases of BCAV, there is a fusion of right and left cusps resulting in right to left systolic opening. In the remaining 20% of cases, there is fusion of right and noncoronary cusps leading to anterioposterior orientation of the valve in systole. These valves with time develop, aortic stenosis or regurgitation or both. Recently, these bicuspid aortic valve patients have been found to have mutations of **NOTCH1**—a gene family. In this condition, there **is failure to inhibit the osteoblastic activity** which leads to calcification early.

- Two thirds develop AS with time, **presenting after the age of 50 years**
- 20% of BCAV develop **aortic regurgitation (AR)**.

- Only 15% of BCAV have normal valve function at 5th decade
- Progression to AS or AR is common with anteroposterior fusion
- They are also prone **to develop IE** at a rate of 0.4 per 1,00,000 per year, which is actually very low
- These persons are also likely to have **dilatation of aorta** unrelated to aortic stenosis
- In a study of young adult with bicuspid valves followed for 9 years from a Canadian center, found that ≥moderate stenosis or ≥moderate regurgitation is a predictor of a composite clinical outcome measure that included hospitalization for heart failure and surgery for valve or aortic disease. The 10-year survival was not different from population estimates for this young population.[2]

Rheumatic AS: Results from adhesions and fusion of the commissures and cusps. Rheumatic AS is always associated with regurgitation of aortic valve and involvement of the mitral valve.

Calcific AS: This is usually occurs after the fourth decade and calcific tricuspid AS is now the most common reason for AS. Such a calcification can occur with bicuspid valves as well. Reason for calcification: Macrophages within lesions produce osteopontin, a protein that modulates calcification. (NEJM Editorial Aug 31, 2000, page 652, JACC August 2003).

Risk factors for calcification are similar to atherosclerosis:

Clinical: Increasing age, male, Hypertension, Diabetes, smoking.

Biochemical: Dyslipedemia, Hyperparathyroidism, Hypercalcemia, Renal failure

In a study from Germany with 10 year follow-up, MONICA/KORA study it was found that Smoking and Cholesterol were the major risk factors for CAVD.[3]

Progression

It has been found that patients with calcific aortic valve disease (CAVD) may progress from risk factors to aortic sclerosis to frank aortic stenosis. This is depicted in the Figure 1. Once these patients become symptomatic, their survival drops down significantly.

HISTORY

Angina: Angina occurs in approximately **two thirds** of patients with severe AS. The chest pain resembles the angina of CAD.

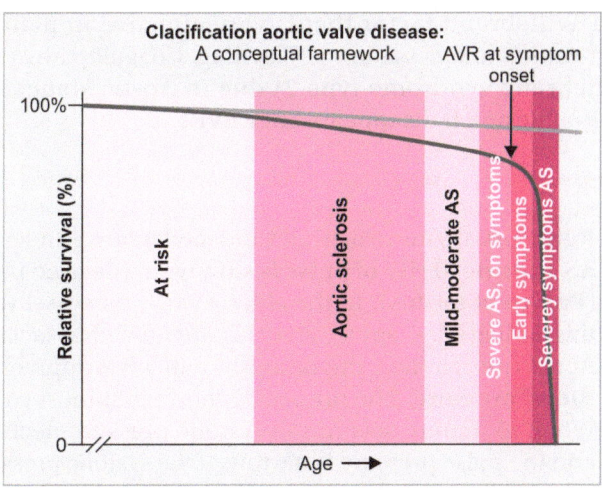

Figure 1 CAVD and progression.
(*Source:* Reproduced with permission from EHJ Aug 2009)

Reasons for Angina

- LVH increases the demand
- Supply is decreased due to prolongation of the LVET, shortening of the diastolic time
- Associated coronary artery disease.
- Calcific emboli to coronary arteries.

Syncope: Syncope can occur either during exertion or at rest.
Effort related syncope can be due to—

- **Fixed cardiac output**: With exercising muscles need more blood causing redistribution of available cardiac output leading to decreased cerebral perfusion and syncope.
- **Baroreceptor mechanism**: Paradoxical forearm vasodilatation due to activation of vagal afferents due to increase in LV end diastolic pressure. This vasodilatation is not accompanied by bradycardia.

Syncope occurring at rest is due to bradycardia or tachycardia, such as ventricle arrhythmias, atrial fibrillation or AV nodal conduction problem (Lev's disease).

Dyspnea: This is a late symptom for patients with AS and if present for more than 5 years, suggests associated mitral valve disease. Filling of thick LV to any given volume requires a higher filling pressure than a ventricle of normal thickness. Hence, the dyspnea is secondary to elevated LVEDP and **diastolic dysfunction.** In addition, these patients develop **systolic dysfunction** with time.

Gastrointestinal bleeding (Heyde Syndrome): Angiodysplasia of the ascending colon has been associated with aortic stenosis. High shear stress due to severe AS increases ADAMTS13 protein in the circulation. This produces an **acquired coagulopathy** by cleaving high molecular weight von-Willebrand factor that is very effective in platelet aggregation and cessation of bleeding. Coagulopathy (von Willebrand syndrome type 2) due to Aortic stenosis is **reversible and it disappears after AVR.**

PHYSICAL FINDINGS

- **Pulse**: Usually normal in mild and moderate AS. In severe AS, **the rate of rise of pulse is slow** with a delayed peak. (**Parvus et tardus**). In the elderly with stiff vessel wall, this finding is less appreciated. In patients with associated Aortic regurgitation, this finding is difficult to appreciate.
- **Blood pressure**: The pressure is normal in most cases. When LV failure sets in the systolic pressure declines and the pulse pressure is narrow. If the systolic pressure is more than 200, then it excludes a severe AS. Between 20–40% with isolated AS may have Systolic BP of 130 mm of HG or more. Hypertension may also be associated with severe AS.[4] Only 6.6% referred for AVR had a pulse **pressure of less than 35 mm Hg**
- **Jugular venous pressure**: Prominent 'a' waves may be seen when the RV cavity shows diminished distensibility to LVH
- **Apical impulse**: The apex is **sustained** with severe AS
- **Systolic Thrill**: Present in the aortic area and in the neck
- **Ejection click**: Aortic ejection click is heard more often with patients of mild stenosis. This sound is often absent in patients with rheumatic aortic stenosis. Aortic ejection sound occurs usually **0.06 seconds** after the first heart sound
- **Ejection systolic murmur** is the most important finding in aortic stenosis. (1). This murmur is **crescendo and decrescendo**, (2). The murmur is low-pitched or **medium pitched,** (3). **Rough and rasping** in quality, (4). Murmur **radiates** to the neck and to apex, (5). The **configuration** of the murmur is useful in assessing the severity of stenosis; with severe AS the murmur tends to peak during the last 60% of systolic. A late peaking murmur occurs when the gradient **is more than 75 mm Hg.** There is a rough correlation between **thrill** and severity of stenosis only in **children;** a grade IV murmur usually indicates that the gradient is more than 50 mm Hg
- Aortic second sound: Aortic component of the S2 is **diminished** in intensity. Paradoxical split of the second heart sound may be present in severe cases. However, clinically it is difficult to make up. **If paradoxical split is present then the gradient is more than 100 mm Hg or LV systolic pressure is more than 160 mm Hg**
- **Dynamic auscultation**

- **Atrial Fib**—The AS murmur **will vary** with Atrial Fib cycle length. This finding will help in differentiating the murmur from systolic murmur of Mitral regurgitation, which does not vary.
- **Squatting:** Murmur is augmented
- **Gallavardian Phenomenon** (Arch Internal Medicine 1974;134:747–9) Gallavardian postulated that the high-pitched musical components of the murmur of aortic stenosis were **preferentially transmitted** to the apex through solid tissues, whereas the lower-pitched components were transmitted to the neck vessels via the flow of blood. Another mechanism for the apical musical murmur has been attributed to associated papillary muscle dysfunction. Third reason which is more often accepted is that the musical component is from the aortic cusps and the murmur heard at the aortic area is from the dilated aorta.

Chest X-ray

- Cardiac size is usually normal; this is because concentric LVH does not cause much cardiac size alteration; cardiomegaly occurs with LV failure
- Ascending aorta may be prominent
- Calcification of the aortic valve can be made out in Fluoroscopy.

ECG

- **LVH** is seen in 85% of patients with severe AS. LVH with **strain** is a **specific marker of mid wall fibrosis** as seen in cMRI. [5]
- **LAE** occurs in 80% of patients with severe AS. This manifests as terminal negativity in lead V1 rather than as increased duration this suggest that hypertrophy is responsible for this finding, rather than dilatation.

Echo Assessment of AS (Table 3)

- Assessment of severity of AS: Peak velocity, Mean gradient and Valve area
- Assessment of other valve lesions
- Quantification of LV systolic function: Ejection fraction, Global longitudinal strain.

Coronary Angiography

Coronary Angiography is done prior to AVR in patients above the age of 35 years to rule out associated coronary artery disease (CAD). Coronary artery disease is present in

Table 3
Parameters to assess aortic stenosis

Parameter	Criteria	Comments
Peak velocity	>4 meters	Easy to obtain Overestimates if aorta is small
Mean gradient	>40 mm Hg	
EOA	<1 sq.cm	Susceptible to measurement errors
Energy Loss Index EOA x Aa/Aa – EOA/BSA	<0.6 cm²/m²	Less flow dependent than gradients Takes into account the pressure recovery Should be measured in all small aorta
Stroke Work Loss 100 x (mean gradient/SBP + Mean gradient)	>25%	Takes into account pressure recovery
Zva = SPB + mean gradient /SVI	>4.5 mm Hgml-1m2	Reflects global load imposd on LV
Aortic valve calification	CT >1650 AU	Correlates with rapid progression
LV EF	<50%	Widely used
Global Longitudinal Strain	<15%	Cutoff values need to be defined Superior to LV EF
Myocardial Fibrosis	cMRI	Predicts poor outcome

Jacc 2012; 60:169-180

25% of patients who do not complain of angina and in 40–80% with angina.

NATURAL HISTORY

- **In Asymptomatic patients**[6]—The rate of progression is related to the baseline velocity as shown in the Table 4.

Table 4
Velocity and rate of progression

Baseline velocity	Rate of progression /year to symptoms
<3 m/sec	8%
2–4	17%
>4	40%

Doppler derived gradients have shown that the gradients increased **for 4–8 mm Hg per year. The aortic valve area decreases by an average of 0.12 sq cm per year.**

Chapter 14: Aortic Stenosis

Predictors of Outcome in Severe Asymptomatic Aortic Stenosis:[7]

In a series of 126 patients with follow-up of 27 months, 8 patients died and 59 patients needed AVR due to symptoms. All of whom had aortic velocity more than 4 m/sec and developed symptoms. The optimal time for surgical intervention is when symptoms develop. **The risk of sudden death is low—1% per year.**

- Asymptomatic LV Dysfunction in aortic Stenosis
    - In one of the largest follow-up series from Mayo clinic of 9940 patients with severe AS it was noted that asymptomatic LV dysfunction was seen in 0.4% of persons.
- Advanced heart failure, reduced ejection fraction and high gradient
    - Prognosis still remains favorable, as long as the mean gradient is more than 40 mm Hg. Thus, no patient should be refused surgery simply because of low EF provided a substantial transvalvular gradient exists.
- Symptoms to death

  Based on the data in patients not treated surgically, **50% survival is** as follows:[8]

  Angina   5 years
  Syncope   3 years
  Dyspnea   2 years
    - **Congestive cardiac failure** is the cause of death in one half to two-thirds of patients. The other cause of death is **sudden death** that occurs in 10-20% of patients at an average of 60 years. However, most sudden deaths occur in patients who are symptomatic.

Table 5

Outcomes in aortic stenosis

	Outcome
Asymptomatic Severe AS, Normal EF	Symptom onset within 3 years in 50–80%
Asymptomatic Severe AS with low EF	EF will normalize with surgery
Symptomatic severe high gradient AS	Mortality is 50% at 1 year, 70–80% in 2 years without AVR
Symptomatic low gradient AS with EF <50%	Mortality at 2 years is 80% with medical and 40% with AVR
Symptomatic low flow, low gradient AS with Normal EF – paradoxical AS	Mortality is 50–70% at 2 years without AVR

Otto NEJM Aug 2014[9]

- **Atrial fibrillation** occurs in 10% of patients in the late stages and worsens the symptoms. This is because the atrial contribution to LV filling is gone and so the cardiac output falls.

SURGERY

Indications for Surgery ACC/AHA 2014[10]

Note that AVR is not routinely recommended for severe AS. (Severe AS is defined as V max of 4 m/s or mean gradient of 40 mm of Hg). The mortality for isolated AVR is around 3–4%. Surgery is indicated only in the following situations.

- Symptomatic—class 1
- Asymptomatic with LV dysfunction EF <50%—class 1
- Severe AS who is undergoing other cardiac surgery—class 1
- Rapid progression—Jet velocity increase is >0.3 m/sec per year—class IIb
- Symptomatic on exercise testing—class 2a (positive test is >2 mm ST depression or failure to increase the systolic BP or fall of BP >20 mm of Hg). It seems reasonable to conclude that a negative exercise test might not require AVR[11]
- Severe AS with Gradient more than 5 meters/sec—Class IIa.

Bicuspid Valve and Aortic Root Surgery (JACC Dec 4, 2015)

- Aortic root or ascending aorta ≥**5.5** cm in size.
- It is *reasonable* in asymptomatic if ascending aorta 5.0-5.5 cm in diameter if an additional risk factor is present for aortic dissection (aortic growth ≥0.5 cm/year or family history of aortic dissection), OR if the patient is at low surgical risk and the surgery is performed by an experienced surgical team.
- In patients with a bicuspid, aortic valve planned for surgical **aortic valve replacement** due to severe aortic stenosis or regurgitation, it is *reasonable* to have a surgical intervention to the ascending aorta if the ascending aorta is >**4.5 cm in size**.

STATINS AND AORTIC STENOSIS PROGRESSION

Aortic stenosis is an active process with many similarities to atherosclerosis. Animal studies and retrospective clinical studies have shown statins to be effective in reducing the progression of aortic stenosis. **Three studies to date have not shown any benefit.**

LOW FLOW LOW GRADIENT AS

- LV ejection fraction less than 40%
- AVA less than 1 sqcm
- Gradient mean <30–40 mm Hg
- Stroke volume index < 35 ml.

Low Dose Dobutamine Echo Test

Usually, dobutamine is given up to a dose of 20 mcg/kg/minute. It is preferable to make each stage as 5 minutes instead of the usual 3 minutes. **MDCT** cut off values for women 1200 and for men 2000 AU (Fig. 2). (Heart 2015: 101:5-6)

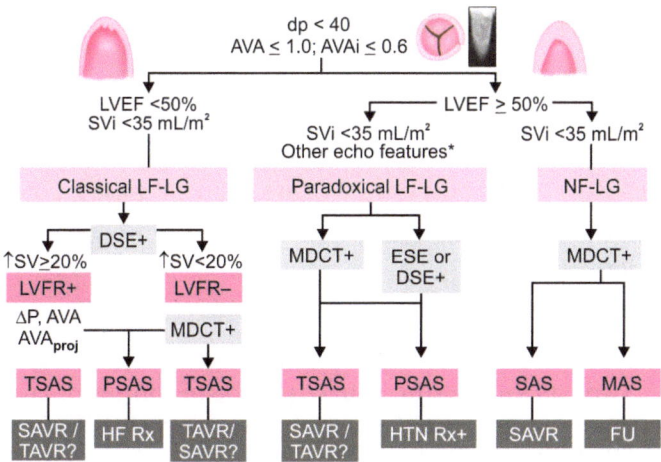

Figure 2 Management of low flow low gradient AS (Circulation Cardiac Imaging May 2014)

AORTIC STENOSIS WITH REGURGITATION

Table 6

Features of combined aortic valve lesion

	Dominant AS	Balanced	Dominant Regurgitation
Syncope	+	+/-	-
Angina	+	+	+
Dyspnea at rest	-	+/-	+
Carotid delay	+	+/-	-
Prolonged systolic Murmur	+	+/-	-
Prolonged diastolic murmur	-	+/-	-
S3	Late	+/-	+ Early
CXR LV dilatation	-	+/-	++

TRANSCATHETER AORTIC VALVE REPLACEMENT – TAVI [12]

TAVR is recommended for Symptomatic severe AS who are at very high risk surgery. The high risk is defined as **STS – PROM score of more than 8**% or irreversible disease of more than two organ systems or possible impediments to a surgical approach.

Indications for Transcatheter AVR – 2014 AHA/ACC Guidelines

- Class 1: Patients who meet an indication for AVR for AS who have a prohibitive surgical risk and a predicted post TAVR survival of more than 12 months
- Class IIa: TAVR is a reasonable alternative to surgical AVR in patients who meet an indication for AVR and who have a high surgical risk.

Table 7
Results of complications of TAVR in randomized trials

	TAVR	Surgery
Stroke	4.9–5.5%	2.4–6.2%
Vascular	5.9–11%	1.7–3.2%
Para valve leak	10–12%	0.9–1.3%
Need for pacemaker	3.8–19.8%	3.6–7%

(*Source:* Otto, NEJM Aug 21, 2014)

Two types of prosthesis have now been approved. They are namely the CoreValve and Edwards SAPIEN valve. In 2002, Cribier et al. did the first human implantation. The aortic valve is approached through the retrograde approach from the femoral artery. Other approach being transapical (hybrid) and antegrade through trans-septal approach.

Differences Between the 2 Approved Valves—CHOICE Trial Data

Sapien valve is a balloon expandable one and the core valve is a self-expanding one. Though the death and stroke rates are similar, it has been noted that the **need for pacemaker and need for re-do valve surgery are higher with the CORE valve Table 8.**

Table 8
CHOICE trial data[13]

	Sapien	Core Valve	p value
30 day mortality %	4.1	5.1	NS
Stroke %	5.8	2.6	NS
Need for Pacemaker %	17.3	37.6	.001
Need for >1 valve %	0.8	5.8	.03

REFERENCES

1. EAE guidelines; European Journal of Echocardiography 2009;10:1-25.
2. Outcomes in adults with bicuspid aortic valves. JAMA. 2008; 300:1317-25.
3. Monica/Kora Study. EHJ. 2009;30(16):2044-53.
4. Das P, Pocock C and Chambers. The patient with systolic murmur: severe AS may be missed during cardiovascular examination. QJM. 2000;93:685-8.
5. Chin et al. Left ventricular hypertrophy and strain in Aortic stenosis. Circulation; 2014.
6. Otto CM. Prospective study of asymptomatic valvular aortic stenosis. Circulation. 1997;95:2262.
7. Rosenhek R. Predictors of Outcome in Severe, asymptomatic aortic stenosis. NEJM. 2000;343:611-7.
8. Ross J and Braunwald E. Aortic Stenosis. Circulation. 1968;38:V-61-7.
9. Otto. Aortic valve stenosis – from patients ar risk to severe valve obstruction. NEJM. 2014;371.
10. Nishimura et al. ACC/AHA guidelines, JACC. March 2014.
11. Dal Bianco et al. Management of asymptomatic severe AS. JACC. October 2008;52:1279-92.
12. Percutaneous aortic valve therapy. Heart. Sept 2009;95: 1538-46.
13. Abdel Waheb M et al. JAMA. 2014;311:1503-14.

CHAPTER 15

Aortic Regurgitation

Jacob Jose

CHAPTER OUTLINE

- Etiology
- Pathophysiology
- Clinical
- Chest X-Ray
- ECG
- Natural History
- Treatment

ETIOLOGY

- Valvular Disease
    - Rheumatic: Cusps infiltrated with fibrous tissue, retract
    - Infective Endocarditis: Perforation/vegetation interfere with valve closure
    - Trauma: Tear/loss of commissural support
    - Bicuspid: Incomplete closure/prolapse
    - Quadricupid: 26% have moderate to severe AR. (Circulation 2015: Dec)
- Aortic Root Disease
    - Annuloaortic ectasia (Idiopathic dilatation)
    - Ankylosing spondylitis
    - Reiters syndrome
    - Psoaritic arthritis
    - Marfans syndrome
    - Osteogenetic imperfecta
    - Rheumatoid arthritis.

Mechanisms of AR in aortic root disease:
- Annulus is dilated
- Cusps become too short to close.

PATHOPHYSIOLOGY

LV Remodeling

- New sarcomeres are added in series and so the individual fibers become longer
- Wall thickness increases as well; more sarcomeres added in parallel also

- Wall stress is increased due to an increase in pressure and volume

Signals for Remodeling

The main source for the remodeling is the **collagen weave** that surrounds the fibers. This collagen weave serves as the wall stress receptor. This is more sensitive to ischemia than are the myocytes and this subendocardial ischemia is probably a major factor in disruption of collagen support system and subsequent fiber layer slippage.

Coronary Flow

Coronary flow reserve is decreased; this occurs due to the following reasons:
- Systolic compression of intramyocardial arteries in hypertrophied arteries
- Perivascular fibrosis
- Low diastolic pressure
- Reversal of flow pattern from diastole to systole.

CLINICAL

- **Palpitations** (increased motion of heart within the chest, that is responsible for the palpitation, rather than the increased force of contraction)
- **Dyspnea:** This is a late symptom and occurs only when there is LV decompensation.
- **Angina**: Often associated with vasoactive phenomena, such as flushing (a pseudo *Nofthnagl* attack). Angina is a result of reduced coronary blood flow that occurs in diastole because of diastolic hypotension. These episodes are more common at night because of the associated bradycardia; with bradycardia, diastole becomes longer and so the degree of AR increases
- Neck pain
- Abdominal pain
- Dizziness.

Arterial Pulse

- Rate per minute — Normal
- Rate of rise — Increased
- Contour of peak — Bisferiens
- Rate of fall — Quick fall
- Systolic pressure — Increased
- Diastolic pressure — Decreased

Peripheral Signs

Head and Neck

- **Corrigan's sign**: Dancing carotids are visible pulsations in both carotid arteries
- **Demusset's sign**: Anterio posterior bobbing of the head
- Beckers's sign: Retinal arteriolar pulsations. This needs close observation in the area in which an arteriole and veins are running closely together and approximately parallel. It is important to note that the retinal venules may pulsate in health but not the arterioles
- **Muller's sign**: Pulsations of Uvula
- Tower house sign (**Oliver–cadarelli's sign**): Alternate redness and pallor of cheeks
- **Ladolfi's sign**: Alternate dilatation and constriction of pupil.

Upper Limb

- **Water Hammer (Corrigan radial)** pulse: The pulse strikes the palpating finger with forceful jerk and quickly disappears (Celer et alter). It is described as having a **water hammer** because of its sudden impact and collapsing quality because it falls away so rapidly.
  - The water hammer effect is accentuated if the pulse is examined by the examiner grasping the hand, and suddenly lifting the hand vertically with his palm. When the patient's hand is suddenly lifted, the radial artery becomes in direct line with the aorta and **the gravity accentuates** the fall of the pulse
  - **Collapsing nature is due to the fact that rapid emptying of the arterial system due to marked increase in the velocity of the blood stream**
  - Pistol shot sound heard over the Water Hammer pulse in the radial would signify severe AR. (NEJM 1952; 247: 771-772)
  - Water Hammer is a Victorian toy that is hermetically sealed with water and exhausted of air.
- **Wide pulse pressure**: More than **50 mm Hg** or 50% of peak systolic pressure
- **Mayne's sign**: Diastolic blood pressure drop of >15 mm of Hg with arm raised
- **Quincke's sign**: This sign may be elicited in several ways
  - Capillary pulsations are observed in the nail bed, when the nail is slightly compressed
  - This can also be observed by pressing a glass slide on inner surface of the lips
  - This sign can be observed by seeing the ear lobe or finger tip while it is being trans illuminated by a torch light

- *Mechanism*: This is due to local dilatation of terminal peripheral vessels.

Lower Limb

- Pistol shot (**Traube's sign**): Auscultation over the femoral artery will reveal a booming sound simultaneous with each pulse. This characteristic sound resembles a pistol shot probably due to vibrations of high frequency caused by sudden elevation of pressure in the vessel
- **Traube's double tone**: Sometimes instead of one sound during systole, two sounds are heard and this is called as Double Tone
- **Duroeziz's** murmur: Diastolic murmur elicited by compressing the stethoscope over the femoral artery. If the murmur is better elicited with distal rim of stethoscope pressure on the artery, then it favors AR. If the murmur is better made out on proximal tilt of the stethoscope it only suggests hyperkinetic flow
- **Hill's sign:** Disproportionate femoral systolic hypertension—the difference between upper limb and lower limb systolic pressure **more than 20 mm Hg.**
  It is **an artifact** of sphygmomanometric lower limb pressure measurement. Hill's sign is the result of the use of inappropriate small size of cuff in the lower limb. With the use of appropriate-sized cuff, Hill' sign is absent in most of the patients with severe AR. If we use intra-arterial pressure measurements, then there **is no difference** between the upper and lower limb blood pressures (Nursing and Midwifery Journal 2008; 4:107-114). If the Hill's sign is more than 60, the AR is noted to be severe. 40–60 mm of Hg is said to be moderate
- **Lincoln sign:** Pulsatile popliteal
- **Sherman sign:** Dorsalis pedis pulse is easily palpable.

Abdomen

- **Rosenbach** sign : Pulsations of the liver
- **Gerhard** sign : Pulsations of the spleen.

Precordial Examination

- Apical impulse: diffuse, hyper dynamic, displaced down and inferiorly
- Rapid filling wave of the left ventricle in severe AR

Auscultation

- Early diastolic murmur
  - EDM is the hallmark of AR. The murmur starts immediately after A2. The duration of the murmur is directly related to the severity in chronic AR.

- Murmur is increased by
    - Squatting
    - Isometric handgrip
    - Inotropic infusion.
- Murmur is decreased by
    - Standing
    - Valsalva strain phase
    - Amyl nitrite inhalation.
- The murmur is best heard with the patient sitting leaning forward and with the breath held in expiration
- Transient arterial occlusion: Both arm are connected to BP apparatus and the cuff is inflated to 20 mm of Hg more than systolic pressure for 20 seconds. If there is an increase in intensity of the murmur, it favors EDM of AR
- Grade 3 murmur also correlates with severe AR. (Desjardins, Am J Med. 1996; 100: 149–156)
- Aortic systolic murmur: The murmur is heard at the base of heart and radiates to neck. However, this murmur is high-pitched and shorter in duration. The murmur is due to increased volume of blood across the aortic valve
- *Mid-diastolic murmur at the mitral area* (Austin Flint murmur).

Mechanism

- The murmur is due to preclosure of mitral valve
- Fluttering of the anterior mitral leaflet due to regurgitant jet impinging on the same
- Diastolic mitral regurgitation due to elevated LV diastolic pressure
- S1 may be diminished in intensity because of preclosure of mitral valve in severe AR, if LV dysfunction is present
- S2 A2 is soft because of poor leaflet coaptation
- S3, if present suggest LV dysfunction
- S4 is heard only in case of acute Aortic regurgitation.

CHEST X-RAY

There is cardiomegaly and the apical impulse is displaced down and out. Ascending aorta may be prominent. Pulmonary congestion is present with LV failure.

ECG

- Left ventiricular hypertrophy (LVH) is common with severe chronic AR. The T waves are upright and tall suggestive of volume overload

Differences between MDM of Mitral stenosis versus Austin flint murmur

	Mitral Stenosis	Austin Flint
S1	Loud	-
S2	P2 loud	-
S3	-	+
LV Enlargement	-	+
RV Enlargement	+	-
Amyl nitrite	+	Decreases
Atrial fibrillation	+	-

- ***LV strain pattern signify advanced LV disease***, such hearts show diminished cardiac contractile reserve and low EF – a marker of chronic subendocardial ischemia.

ECHO–ESC guidelines 2013—Grading of the severity of AR[1]

Parameters	*Mild*	*Moderate*	*Severe*
Qualitative			
Aortic valve morphology	Normal/abnormal	Normal/abnormal	Abnormal/flail/large Coaptation defect
Color flow AR jet width	Small in central jets	Intermediate	Large in central jet, variable in eccentric jets
CW signal of AR jet	Incomplete/faint	Dense	Dense
Diastolic flow reversal in the descending aorta	Brief, protodiastolic flow reversal	Intermediate	Holodiastolic flow reversal (end-diastolic velocity >20cm/s)
Semiquantitative			
VC width (mm)	<3	Intermediate	6
Pressure half-time (ms)	>500	Intermediate	<200
Quantitative			
EROA (mm2)	<10	Intermediate values	>30
R Vol (mL)	<30	Intermediate values	>60

NATURAL HISTORY

Death occurs **within 4 years** after the development of angina and **within 2 years** after the onset of heart failure.

10 year follow-up in Rheumatic Aortic Regurgitation[2]

In a study done in Brazil, they followed 75 patients with severe aortic regurgitation, age 28 ± 9 years over a period of 10 ± 0.69 years. 37 patients developed symptoms and 38 patients remained asymptomatic and were managed medically. Multivariate analysis showed that the probability of developing symptoms within 10 years was 58% for a patient with LVID(d) >70 mm and 76% for a patient with LVID(s) >50 mm. The overall survival was 90% for a 10-year followup. *The need for AVR can be based on the symptoms rather than specific values of LV dimensions* in Rheumatic aortic regurgitation.

Natural History of Aortic Regurgitation:[3]

1. **Asymptomatic with Normal LV function:**

Progression to symptoms / LV dysfunction	**6% year**
Progression to Asymptomatic LV dysfunction	3.5% year
Sudden death	0.2% year

2. **Asymptomatic with LV dysfunction:**

Progression to Symptoms	25% year

3. **Symptomatic patients**

Mortality	10% year

TREATMENT

Vasodilators

The main goal of drug therapy with vasodilators is to reduce the systolic hypertension associated with severe chronic Aortic Regurgitation, and thereby reduce the wall stress and improve LV function.[4]

- Vasodilators, such as Nifedipine be given for patients **Severe AR and systolic blood pressure more than 140** mm Hg or so with normal LV function
- Vasodilators may be considered for patients with **severe AR and LV dilatation** but without LV systolic dysfunction
- The other group we can give is the group of patients of **AR with LV dysfunction** on a **short-term** before proceeding for AVR[5]
- Vasodilator therapy is **not indicated** of asymptomatic patients with mild or moderate AR or for long-term in patients with severe AR and LV dysfunction.

Indications for Surgery in Severe AR (ACC/AHA June 2014)[6]

- Symptomatic severe AR (class 1)
- Asymptomatic severe AR with EF less than 50% (class 1)
- Asymptomatic severe AR going for other cardiac surgery (class 1)
- Asymptomatic with LV dimension in systole >50 mm (class 2a)
- Asymptomatic with LV dimension in diastole >65 mm (class 2b).

Recommendations for Angiogram in severe AR:

- For the assessment of coronaries before aortic valve replacement
- Assessment severity of AR, when noninvasive tests are inconclusive or discordant with clinical findings.

REFERENCES

1. ESC guidelines EHJ–cardiovascular Imaging. 2013;14:611-44.
2. Tarasoutchi F, Grinberg M, Spina GS, et al. Ten year clinical laboratory follow-up of after application of a system based therapeutic strategy to patients with severe chronic aortic regurgitation of predominant rheumatic etiology. JACC. 2003; 41:1316-24.
3. ACC/AHA guidelines for the management of patients with valvular heart disease. JACC. 1998;32:1486-1588.
4. Bekeredjian R, Grayburn PA. Valvular Heart Disease: Aortic Regurgitation. Circulation. 2005;112:125-134.
5. RobertsWC, et al. Valvular Heart Disease: Causes of pure aortic regurgitation in patients having isolated aortic valve replacement at a single US tertiary hospital (1993 to 2005). Circulation. 2006;114:422-9.
6. ACC/AHA guidelines. 2014;63:e57-e185.

CHAPTER 16

Mitral Stenosis

Jacob Jose

CHAPTER OUTLINE

- Etiology
- Hemodynamics
- Atrial Fibrillation
- Auscultation
- Chest X-Ray
- ECG
- Natural History
- Juvenile Ms

ETIOLOGY

- Rheumatic—Commonest
- Congenital—Less frequent
- Rarely:
  - Rheumatoid
  - SLE
  - Hunter-Hurler
  - Malignant carcinoid
  - Methysergide therapy.

Mechanism of Production of Mitral Stenosis in Rheumatic Fever

- Fusion of the mitral valve apparatus
- Commissural   30%
- Cuspal   15%
- Chordae   10%
- All of the above   45%.

HEMODYNAMICS

Severity of mitral stenosis in relation to valve area is shown in Table 1

Table 1
Severity of mitral stenosis in relation to valve area

Severity	Valve area (sq.cm)	Pressure half time (m.sec)
Mild	2	
Moderate	1.5 to 2	Less than 150
Severe	<1.5	150
Very severe	<1	220

(ACC/AHA, JACC June 2014)

Valve Area and Gradients

At a MVA of 1 cm^2, the mitral diastolic gradient to maintain normal cardiac output at rest is around 20 mm Hg. The Table 2 shows the relation between valve area and gradients.

Table 2
Severity of mitral stenosis in relation to gradient

Severity	Gradient mm of Hg
Mild	<5
Moderate	5–10
Severe	>10

Features of LA Pressure Tracing

- Mean LA pressure increased
- Slow Y descent
- Prominent 'a' wave.

Pulmonary Hypertension

- The pulmonary hypertension in mitral stenosis can be of two types:
  - Passive
  - Reactive does not occur unless the LA mean is at least 20 mm of Hg.
- PH is common in Mitral stenosis than in isolated mitral regurgitation. The reason being that diastole is approximately two thirds of cardiac cycle, LV diastolic pressure or LA pressure is transmitted to the pulmonary veins for relatively longer period than is systolic pressure. Hence, diseases that elevate the **diastolic pressures are more often likely** to be associated with secondary PH than are diseases that cause isolated elevation of systolic pressure[1]
- **Reactive PH** means that the transpulmonary gradient is more than 10 mm of Hg, i.e. PA mean – PA wedge (LA mean)
- At a PA pressure of 70 mm Hg or more, the RV failure is manifest
- ***Jordans Hypothesis:*** Alveolar wall thickening, fibrosis, hypoventilation of the lower lobes, hypoxemia of the lower lobe pulmonary veins, chemoreceptors of PV causes PA arteriolar constriction and hence, reactive PH.

ATRIAL FIBRILLATION[2]

History

- ***Dyspnea:*** This symptom is due to pulmonary congestion leading onto reduced pulmonary complaints. This is the most prominent symptom of MS.

Table 3
Relationship between age and atrial fibrillation

Age in years	Incidence %
11–20	0
21–30	17
31–40	45
41–50	60
>51	80

- ***Hemoptysis:*** There are several reasons for the same and they are given below: (a) Acute pulmonary edema, (b) Paraxysmal nocturnal dyspnea, (c) Pulmonary infarction, (d) Bronchitis, (e) Pulmonary apoplexy—due to rupture of small bronchial vein
- ***Chest pain:*** It is observed in less than 15% of patients and clinically resembles angina due to coronary artery disease. (a) Right ventricular ischemia secondary to pulmonary hypertension, (b) Associated coronary artery disease c. Coronary embolism
- ***Hoarseness of voice (ORTNER syndrome):*** Sengupta et al. concluded that the etiology of left recurrent laryngeal nerve paralysis was compression of the nerve between the **enlarged tense left pulmonary artery and the aorta at the ligamentum arteriosum**. That is the reason why Ortner syndrome may also occur in primary pulmonary hypertension, Eisenmenger syndrome due to atrial septal defect where the left atrium is not enlarged, and even aortic aneurysms with encroachment of aorticopulmonary window and resultant compression of the left recurrent laryngeal nerve can happen[3]
- ***Embolic manifestations:*** Patients with MS are prone to develop embolic manifestations. There is a direct correlation between age of the patient, left atrial size and rhythm of the patient in developing embolism. More than 50% of all emboli lodge in cerebral vessels. Emboli are recurrent in 25% of patients.

Table 4
Relationship between age, rhythm and systemic embolism[4]

Age	Rhythm	Embolism %
<35	SR	5
>35	SR	11
<35	A fib	27
>35	A fib	32

AUSCULTATION

In mitral stenosis, there are four important auscultatory findings:
1. Loud first heart sound
2. Opening snap
3. Mid-diastolic murmur
4. Presystolic murmur

Loud First Heart Sound

S1 is Loud for the following Reasons

- Elevated LA pressure in late diastole that allows LV pressure to rise higher than normal before LV-LA cross over
- **Wide closing excursion** of the mitral leaflets
- Stiff noncompliant leaflets resonate with an increased sound amplitude.

Loudness and Calcification

A loud first heart sound indicates that the valve is pliable and it is noncalcific. When the valve is calcified the first heart sound may be comes off. Calcification limited to the posterior mitral leaflet will not alter the loudness of the first heart sound if the body of the anterior mitral leaflet is mobile.

Opening Snap

- Sudden tensing of the leaflets after the valve cusps have completed their opening excursion
- The interval between second and OS is the sum of true Isovolumic relaxation time plus mitral valve excursion
- The narrow 2-OS interval and long is shown in the Table 5.

Table 5
S2 - OS interval

Narrow 2–OS interval	Long
Less than 0.08 sec	More than 0.10
MS tight	MS mild
Tachycardia	Hypertension—aortic systolic BP >130, 2-OS is unreliable
	Bradycardia
	Poor LV function
	Aortic regurgitation
	Low LA pressure due to large LA

A short 2-OS interval is more reliable than large 2-OS interval because there are several reasons for a long interval (Table 6).

Table 6
S2-OS interval and its relationship to the severity of mitral stenosis[5]

Severity	S2-OS interval
Mild	100–120 msec
Moderate	80–100 msec
Severe	<80 msec

Differentiating A2–P2 from 2 OS

- Standing: 2-OS widens
- Inspiration: triple sound; 2-OS widens
- Exercise: 2-OS shortens.

Causes of soft OS in Mitral Stenosis
- Calcific valve
- Low flow
- AR severe.

Mid Diastolic Murmur

This is the third auscultatory feature of mitral stenosis
- *Site:* Best heard at the apex
- *Pitch:* Low-pitched *conduction:* None, localized
- *Character:* Rough and rumbling
- *Loudness:* May be associated with thrill
- *Exercise:* The murmur increases
- *Posture:* The murmur is best heard in the left lateral position and decreases during standing
- *Valsalva:* The murmur may disappear or decrease in intensity
- *Respiration:*
  - With inspiration, sometimes the heart rate increases and the murmur may get exaggerated (false positive CARVALLO's sign)
  - Usually the murmur is best heard in expiration because of increasing venous return.

Differential Diagnosis of Mid-Diastolic Murmur

- **Carey Coombs Murmur:** This is the short mid-diastolic murmur heard in acute rheumatic fever. S1 is not loud and this murmur is never associated with the thrill. It is recognized by the company it keeps. It is always associated with MR murmur
- **Left Atrial Myxoma:** The murmur varies with positional changes. In addition, there will be a Tumor plop
- **Austin Flint Murmur (AFM):** This murmur is present in patients with severe aortic regurgitation. The differentiating points are given in Table 7.

Table 7
Differences between mitral MDM and austin Flint murmur

		Mitral stenosis	Austin flint murmur
1	S1 loud	Present	No
2	P2 loud	Present	Rare
3.	S3	Never	May be present
4	Opening snap	Present	No
5	Amyl nitrate	Murmur Increases	Murmur decreases
6	Rhythm	May be AFib	Sinus rhythm
7	Peripheral signs of AR	None	Present
8	Apex beat	Tapping	Hyperdynamic

Presystolic Murmur (PSM)

- This murmur is heard in the patients with mitral stenosis if the pressure gradient exceeds 3 mm Hg at least in the end diastole
- Though it is absent in atrial fibrillation, can be present in patients with severe MS
- Mechanism—
    - Atrial contraction increases the gradient
    - LV contraction in presystole reduces the mitral funnel.
- PSM may be absent in—
    - Mild MS
    - AFib
    - Prolonged PR
    - Elevated LVEDP
    - Bradycardia.

Table 8
Auscultatory features of severity of MS

Severity of MS	2-OS interval msec	Murmur
Mild	100–120	Short MDM or PSM only
Moderate	80–100	MDM + PSM with a gap
Severe	Less than 80	MDM +PSM without a gap

CHEST X-RAY

Cardiac silhouette
- L A E
- PA prominent
- RV and RA enlargement

Lung fields
- Kerley B lines
- Kerley A lines
- Upper lobe veins are prominent—Antler's sign
- Pulmonary hemosiderosis
- Pulmonary ossification

ECG

- Left Atrial Enlargement
  - LAE P mitrale—widened P in Lead 2 is the most consistent sign.
  - P terminal force—biphasic p wave with negativity – the negative area more than 0.04 is called as **Morris index**
- RVH
  - If the RVSP is 70–100, then 50% have ECG RVH
  - If RVSP >100 all most all have ECG RVH.
- RAD
  - If the axis is more than 60, the valve area is less than 1.3 sq cm.
- Atrial fibrillation—If coarse AFib, it is a sign of LAE.

NATURAL HISTORY

It usually takes 5–10 years for patients to progress from mild to severe symptoms. In countries like India, the progression can be more rapid and critical mitral stenosis can be present in children as early as 6 years of age.

In one study from Greece, the mean interval from acute RF to appearance of symptoms was 16.3 + 5.2 years and progression of mild to severe disability was 9.2 ± 4.3 years on an average.

Two echo follow-up studies suggest that the valve area decreases on average of 0.09 cm^2/year

MANAGEMENT

- Rheumatic fever prophylaxis
- Infective endocarditis prophylaxis not required
- Drugs to control pulmonary congestion—diuretics
- Rate reducing drugs such as beta blocker/verapamil
- Balloon mitral valvotomy (BMV/PTMC) or mitral valve replacement
- **Anticoagulation:** The indications are as follows—**5 in total**. (i) Atrial Fib (Class 1), (ii) Prior embolic episode even in sinus rhythm (Class 1), (iii) LA thrombus (Class 1), (iv) LA dimension >55 mm—Class 2b, (v) Large LA with spontaneous echo contrast—class 2 b

PTMC/BMV Indications (ACC/AHA - JACC June 2014)

- Symptomatic with MVA less than 1.5—class 1
- Asymptomatic with MVA less than 1sq.cm—class 2a
- Asymptomatic with new onset Atrial Fib and MVA less than 1.5 sq.cm—class 2b
- Progress MS (MVA >1.5sqcm but with exercise the wedge pressure is more than 25 mm of Hg—class 2b.

Chapter 16: Mitral Stenosis

Absolute Contraindications for PTMC

- LA thrombus
- More than mild MR
- Severe mitral valve calcification especially the commissures
- Contraindications for transeptal puncture
- Cardiothoracic deformity
- Bleeding disorders.

BMV may increase the degree of MR by one grade in 30% and by 2 grades in 15%. Therefore, patients with 2 + or greater usually are not recommended for BMV.

Relative Contraindications for PTMC

- Echo score 10 or more
- Thick atrial septum >3 mm
- Severe subvalvar fibrosis.

Results of PTMC from India

- **George Joseph** has summarized the complications bserved in the series from CMC Hospital, Vellore.[6]

– Death	0.5%
– Cardiac tamponade	0.6%
– Severe MR	2.6%
– MVR	0.9%
– Stroke, TIA	0.1%

- **Arora** et al.[7] reported their data in a group of 4,850 patients. The mortality was 0.2%, cardiac tamponade 0.2%, embolism 0.1%, mitral regurgitation severe 1.4%, **restenosis was observed in 4.8% of these patients** on a 94-month follow-up.
- **Manjuanth** et al. from Jayadeva have published their experience in more than 12,000 PTMC and theirs' is the largest so far.[8]

Restenosis after PTMC

- In the Arora series, the restenosis rate was 4.8% at 94 months.

Effect of PTMC and Atrial Fibrillation[9]

BMV as a favorable effect on the incidence of atrial fibrillation. In one study from Saudi Arabia, the incidence was 8.9% in the follow-up after BMV versus 29% in patients without BMV.

20 year Results of PTMC (Circulation 2012; 125: 2119 – 2127)

30% of patients at 20 years were in good functional result—defined as survival without mitral surgery or repeat PTMC and in NYHA class I or II.

JUVENILE MS

Dr Roy published an article in Lancet in the year 1963, the clinical and physiopathological findings of 108 patients with mitral stenosis who were below the age of 20 years. The following points are noteworthy:
- Two-thirds of had mean PA pressure elevated
- The pulmonary artery branches accompanying terminal and respiratory bronchios and arterioles showed pronounced medial muscular hypertrophy
- There was smooth muscle cell proliferation of distal air passages.

ECHO Approach to Mitral Stenosis

- To assess the severity of mitral stenosis
- Associated mitral regurgitation
- Associated other valve lesions
- PA pressure estimation from TR
- Valve suitability for BMV.

Table 9

Wilkins' echo score used to predict outcome in BMV

Grade	Mobility	Subvalvar thickening	Thickening	Calcification
1	Leaflet tip is restricted	Just below leaflets	Leaflets near normal in thickness	A single area
2	Mid and base have normal mobility	Up to one third of the chordal length	Mid leaflets normal, marked thickening of margins, 5–8 mm	Scattered area confined to leaflet margins
3	Base only has normal mobility	Distal third of chords	Entire leaflet is thickened, 5–8 mm	Mid portion
4	No or minimal	Extends up to papillary muscle	Marked thickness > 8 mm	Throughout

Left Atrial Clot

LA clot has been observed in **6.6% of patients with Sinus Rhythm** as well. The predictors for this age are more than 44 years or LA inferosuperior dimension more than 69 mm or dense spontaneous echo-contrast.[10] A classification of the LA clot is given below in the Figure 1.

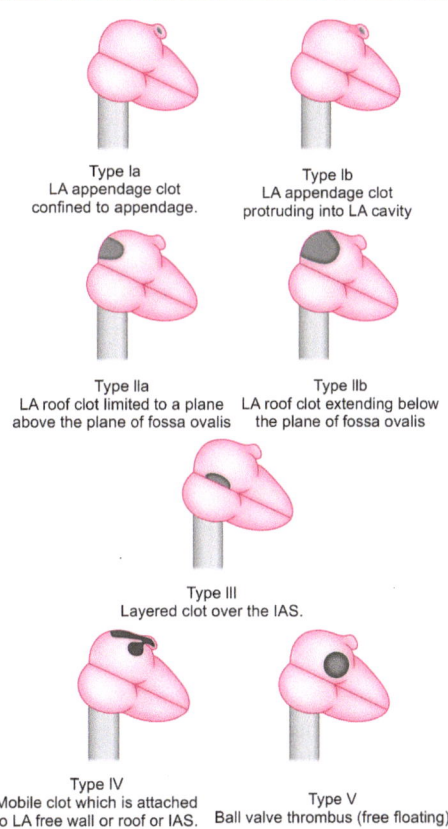

Figure 1 LA clot classification in mitral stenosis (Manjunath et al.)

REFERENCES

1. Feigenbaum' Echocardiography, Chapter 6, page 169, 6th Edition.
2. Deverall PB et al. Incidence of systemic embolism before and after mitral valvotomy. Thorax. 1968;23:530.
3. Sengupta et. J of Layrn and Otology. 1998;112:377-9.
4. Coulshed N, et al. Systemic embolism in mitral valve disease. Br. Heart J 1970; 32:36
5. Carabello. Modern management of mitral stenosis. Circulation. 2005;112:432-8.
6. Jomiva Balloon Catheter Instruction Manual, second edition 2002: 23-24
7. Arora et al. Results of Balloon Mitral Valvotomy. Cardiac Catheter Interventions 2002; 55: 450-456.
8. Manjunath et al. Mitral Valve disease, Medicine Update. 2010;20:368-74
9. Fawzy M E, et al. Favorable effect of balloon mitral valvuloplasty on the Incidence of atrial fibrillation in patients with severe mitral stenosis. Catheterization and Cardiovascular interventions. 2006;68:536-41.
10. Manjunath et al. Incidence and predictors for LA thrombus. Echocardiography, 2011;28:457-60.

CHAPTER 17

Mitral Regurgitation

Jacob Jose

CHAPTER OUTLINE

- Etiology
- Types of MR
- Clinical Examination
- Echo Grading of Severity - ESC 2013 Guidelines
- Natural History
- Surgery
- Mitral Valve Repair
- Medical Treatment for Primary MR

ETIOLOGY

- Rheumatic heart disease
- Mitral valve prolapse
- Infective endocarditis
- Dilated cardiomyopathy
- Ischemic heart disease
- Congenital: Cleft mitral leaflet, endocardial cushion defect.

TYPES OF MR

- Type 1: Normal leaflet motion—Ischemic MR, DCM
- Type 2: Increased leaflet motion—Marfan's, Fibroelastic deficiency, Barlow disease
- Type 3a: Restricted leaflet motion with restricted opening—Rheumatic, carcinoid, SLE, Ergotamine use
- Type 3b: Restricted leaflet motion—Restrictive closure: Ischemic Cardiomyopathy or Dilated CMY.

CLINICAL EXAMINATION

Precordial Examination

- LV impulse is **hyperdynamic** with a normal contour and increased amplitude of early systolic outward motion
- **Late systolic** parasternal lift (Fig. 1)
- **Parasternal** heave of RVH.

Heart Sounds

- *First heart sound:* The most frequent abnormality is a decrease in S1 amplitude

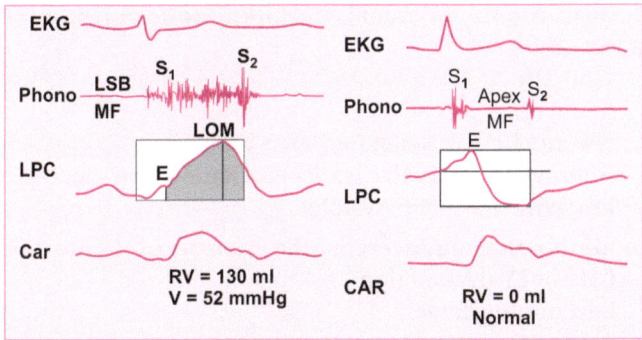

Figure 1 Shown above is the recording of the parasternal movement in a patient with MR severe and on the left of a normal person. Note the late outward movement on the left figure reaches its peak in late systole. A ratio can be calculated for the LOM and the E wave which correlates with the severity of MR.[1]

- *Second sound:* In severe cases, it is audibly split in expiration, because of a shortened LV ejection time
- *Third heart sound:* Is common in MR of hemodynamic significance; it does not indicate LV dysfunction
- *Fourth heart sound:* is **never a feature** of it rheumatic mitral valve disease. The LA of chronic MR any etiology is dilated and compliant and is unable to generate an atrial sound or S4. In acute MR, it can produce S4.

MR Murmur

It is systolic murmur best heard in the mitral area with one of the following configurations.
- Holo systolic with plateau configuration
- Late systolic accentuation
- Late systolic taper
- Mid systolic accentuation—Ejection systolic murmur

Murmur of Rheumatic MR

- In RHD, the most common variant is mid or late systolic accentuation of the murmur. In more severe MR, murmur is more likely to have a mid systolic accentuation giving it a spindle-shaped or ejection quality. In all these situations, careful auscultation usually will identify sound vibrations at the beginning and at end systole, which confirm that the murmur is truly regurgitant in quality as opposed to a more common ejection systolic murmur
- Usually, it is conducted to left axilla and back and this is due to the fact that the regurgitant jet is directed posterolaterally.

The least common variant is the **late systolic murmur**. The causes are:
- Mild MR
- Acute MR
- Severe MR in to small LA (large V wave)
- Improved mitral valve leaflet coaptation from decreased LV cavity size in late systole.

Conditions that may decrease the intensity of MR murmur:
- CHF or LV dysfunction
- Low output states
- Associated MS
- Huge LA
- Obesity, thick chest wall, etc.

Bedside clues to significant MR:
- Rhythm—Atrial fibrillation
- Carotid pulse—small volume quick rising
- LV impulse
- LA impulse
- S2 wide split
- S3 present
- Murmur very loud and widely conducted. The correlation between loudness and severity is deceptive since it will depend on the LV pressure and LV function and the etiology.

Maneuvers

- **Left Decubitus position:** Will usually **augment the murmur of MR** and often increase its intensity by one to two grades. In addition this maneuver occasionally accentuates the holosystolic murmur of a late systolic tapering murmur. Use this position when an apical murmur is low amplitude and long duration.
- **Standing:** May decrease or no change in Rheumatic MR. If due to MVP then it may increase.
- **Valsalva:** Rheumatic MR will decrease and MVP MR will increase
- **Phenylephrine:** In MVP, it will decrease the murmur due to reflex bradycardia and increase in the LV cavity size
- **Respiration:** No change.

Thrill

Usually, MR murmur is only grade 3 or less. Thrill is less common with MR. If present then we need to think of associated conditions such as
- Chordal rupture
- Infective endocarditis
- Aortic stenosis or VSD murmur is mistaken for MR murmur.

Table 1
Dynamic auscultation

Intervention	Hypertrophic Obstructive Cardiomyopathy	Aortic Stenosis	Mitral regurgitation	Mitral valve prolapse
Valsalva	↑	↓	↓	↑ or ↓
Standing	↑	↑ or unchanged	↓	↑
Handgrip or Squatting	↓	↓ or unchanged	↑	↓
Supine position with legs elevated	↓	↑ or unchanged	Unchanged	↓
Exercise	↑	↑ or unchanged	↓	↑
Amyl nitrite	↑↑	↑	↓	↑
Isoproterenol	↑↑	↑	↓	↑

ECHO GRADING OF SEVERITY – ESC 2013 GUIDELINES[2]

The grading of mitral regurgitation severity is being given in Table 2.

NATURAL HISTORY

- 80% survival at 5 years and 60% survival at 10 years after the diagnosis
- Patients with combined Mitral stenosis and Mitral regurgitation have a poor prognosis and only 30% survival at 10 years
- Flail leaflet: Incidence on a 10-year follow-up:
  Atrial fibrillation   30%
  Congestive Heart Failure   60%
  Surgery or death   90%

Table 2
Grading of mitral regurgitation severity

	Mild	Moderate	Severe
Specific signs of severity	• Small central jet <4cm² or <20% of LA area • Vena contracta width <0.3cm • No or minimal flow convergence	Signs of MR >mild present, but no criteria for severe MR	• Vena contracta width ≥0.7cm with large central MR jet (area>40% of LA) or with a wall a imcpinging in LA

Contd...

Contd...

	Mild	Moderate	Severe
			• Large flow convergence • Systolic reversal in pulmonary veins • Prominent flail MV leaflet or ruptures papillary muscle
Supportive signs	• Systolic dominant flow in pulmonary veins • A wave dominant mitral inflow • Soft density, parabolic CW Doppler MR signal • Normal LV size	Intermediate signs/findings	• Dense, triangular CW Doppler MR jet • E-wave dominant mitral inflow (E>1.2m/s) Enlarged LV and LA size
Quantitative parameters R Vol (ml/beat) RF (%) EROA (cm2)	<30 <30 <0.20	30-44 45-59 30-39 40-49 0.20-0.29 0.30-0.39	≥60 ≥50 ≥0.40

■ SURGERY

Indications for surgery—ACC/AHA guidelines 2014[3]
- Symptomatic severe MR—class 1
- Asymptomatic severe MR with LV dysfunction (LVIDs >40 mm or EF 30 to 60%) Class 1. This is called as 60/40 rule
- Asymptomatic severe MR if **repair is likely** with a mortality is less than 1% with LV function Normal (EF >60% and LVIDs <40mm—class 2a. New onset A Fib OR PASP more than 50 mm of Hg
- Symptomatic severe primary MR with LVEF less than 30% Class 2b
- For secondary MR: MVR may be considered for symptomatic class 3 or 4 (class 2b): MV repair—moderate MR if other cardiac surgery is being undertaken—class 2b.

MITRAL VALVE REPAIR

- The operative mortality is much less compared to Mitral valve replacement (1.6%)
- Postoperative embolism and endocarditis is much lower when compared to MVR
- Feasibility of Mitral valve repair depends on the etiology and this is summarized in the table below

Table 3
Mitral valve repair success

Mechanism	Repair success rate
Posterior chordal rupture–Myxomatous	80%
Anterior chordal rupture–Myxomatous	63%
Anterior and posterior chordal rupture	40%
Rheumatic	45–50%
Endocarditis	45–50%
Elongated chordae	81%

Predictors of Recurrent Functional MR after Annuloplasty

Numerous preoperative predictors of recurrent secondary MR after undersized annuloplasty have been identified and are indicative of severe tethering, and associated with a worse prognosis.
- LVIDd more than 65 mm
- Posterior mitral leaflet angle >45
- Distal anterior mitral leaflet angle>.25
- Systolic tenting area >2.5 cm^2
- Coaptation distance (distance between the annular plane and the coaptation point) >10 mm
- End-systolic interpapillary muscle distance >.20 mm, and
- Systolic sphericity index >0.7.

MEDICAL TREATMENT FOR PRIMARY MR

- ACE group of drugs have not shown to be of benefit unless there is heart failure
- Beta-blockers have also not shown to benefit based on retrospective and small prospective trials
- RF prophylaxis is indicated for RHD
- Diuretics are given for pulmonary congestion.

REFERENCES

1 Basta et al. The value of para sternal recordings in the assessment of Mitral regurgitation. Circulation. Nov 1973; 48:1055-65.
2 Echo guidelines: European Heart Journal of Imaging. 2013;14:611-44.
3 Nishimura et al. 2014 AHA /ACC guidelines. JACC. 2014; 63: e57-185.

CHAPTER 18

Prosthetic Valve

Jacob Jose

CHAPTER OUTLINE

- Case scenario
- Types of valves
- Auscultation
- Anticoagulation
- Mechanical or tissue valve aortic homograft
- Investigations
- Complications
- Excessive anticoagulation
- Bridging therapy
- Coronary angiogram before valve surgery
- Heart Failure after valve replacement
- AFib ablation during mitral valve replacement
- TAVI or TAVR

CASE SCENARIO

60-year-old male who had undergone MVR with St Jude Mitral valve 5 years ago, now presents with increasing dyspnea, gradual onset, now in NYHA class 3. He is only on warfarin and he has not been checking blood PT INR regularly. On examination, he has elevated JVP, short systolic murmur over the mitral area and prosthetic sounds are heard. Liver is palpable 4 fingers below coastal margin.

TYPES OF VALVES

Prosthetic valves can be classified into 2 types, namely Mechanical and Tissue valve.

Mechanical

1. Ball and cage – Starr–Edwards, discontinued in 2007.
2. Tilting disk – Medtronic/Sri Chitra.
3. Bileaflet – St.Jude, ATS, On X.

Tissue

These valves once endothelialized do not require anticoagulation unless patient has another indication for the same. Hence, anticoagulation is given **only for the first 3 months**. However, if the patient has atrial fibrillation then the patient should continue anticoagulation.

1. **Stented bioprostheses**
   Heterografts: Porcine—Carpentier edwards, hancock – heterografts,
   Bovine: Pericardial—Carpentier edwards pericardial – heterografts
2. **Stentless Bioprostheses**
   Toronto
   Medtronic free style
3. **Transcatheter Bioprostheses**
4. **Allografts** (**Homografts**): Cadaveric aortic valve
5. **Autografts**
   Ross procedure: Patients' own pulmonary valve is used to replace the aortic valve. In the pulmonary position, an aortic homograft is placed – aortic valve taken from a cadaver.
   Pericardial Autografts: Patients own pericardium is inserted into a frame and is used in the aortic position. Long term durability is excellent especially in the elderly.
6. **Tissue engineered heart valves (TEHV)**[1]
   Autologous bone marrow derived mononuclear cells are integrated into nitinol stents have been studied in sheep models.

AUSCULTATION

The auscultatory features of these valves are summarized in the Figure 1.
- Any diastolic murmur in the aortic position and any holo systolic murmur in the mitral position are **abnormal**.
- Decreased intensity of the closing clicks is abnormal.
- If the valve is of the **ball and cage type** then the opening and closing clicks are prominent.
- If the valve is of the **tilting disk type, then closing click is prominent** and the opening click is not prominent.

ANTICOAGULATION

All prosthetic valves require oral anticoagulation to prevent embolism. Mechanical valves require oral anticoagulation for life and for tissue valves for a short time as given below. The commonly used oral anticoagulation drugs are Vitamin K antagonists such as **Warfarin or Acenocoumarol** (Acitrom).

Mechanical Valves

- The target INR is 2-3 for aortic position and for mitral 2.5 to 3.5 – life long.
- Aspirin in addition 75 mg per day.

Tissue Valves

- Mitral – Warfarin for 3 months and aspirin thereafter.
- Aortic – Warfarin for 3 months and aspirin thereafter.

Risk of Bleeding with Warfarin

- Minor – 2–4% per year
  Major – 1–2% per year
  Death – 0.2–0.4% per year due to bleeding.

MECHANICAL OR TISSUE VALVE – ACC/AHA JUNE 2014

1. Tissue valve may be recommended for patients who have a **contraindication to taking warfarin** – class Ic indication
2. Tissue valves are recommended for patients **above the age of 70 years** – class IIa.
3. Mechanical valves if age is < 60 years—class IIa.
4. Either a Mechanical or Tissue valve in patients between 60 years and 70 years of age—class IIa.

Randomized Studies on Mechanical Versus Tissue Valves

1. VA study: 575 patients follow-up of 15 years, mitral valve degeneration noted at 5 years and 7 years for aortic valve for tissue valves.
2. Edinberg Heart valve trial: 541 patients followed up for 20 years, event free survival better with mechanical valve.

AORTIC HOMOGRAFT

This valve is of choice in **aortic valve endocarditis. The reason being that infection rate is low.** The surgery requires re-implantation of coronary arteries and these valves do calcify with time. So if a re-operation is required, then it will be technically demanding.

INVESTIGATIONS

1. **Echo Doppler** (JASE Sept 2009): This is the most important investigation for the follow-up of patients after prosthetic valve implantation. Each patient should have his **base-line values** before discharge following surgery. If the baseline value was done before discharge, we do it within 1 month of surgery. This will form the reference guide in the follow up. TEE is required for the complete evaluation of mitral prosthetic valve.
   - **Mitral Valve:** If the velocity gradient across the valve is > 2.5 m/sec or pressure half time (PHT) > 200 msec, it is abnormal (Table 18.1).
   - **Aortic valve: Peak velocity more than 4 m/sec is abnormal.** All prosthetic valves are inherently obstructive and so gradient across it is common (Table 18.2).

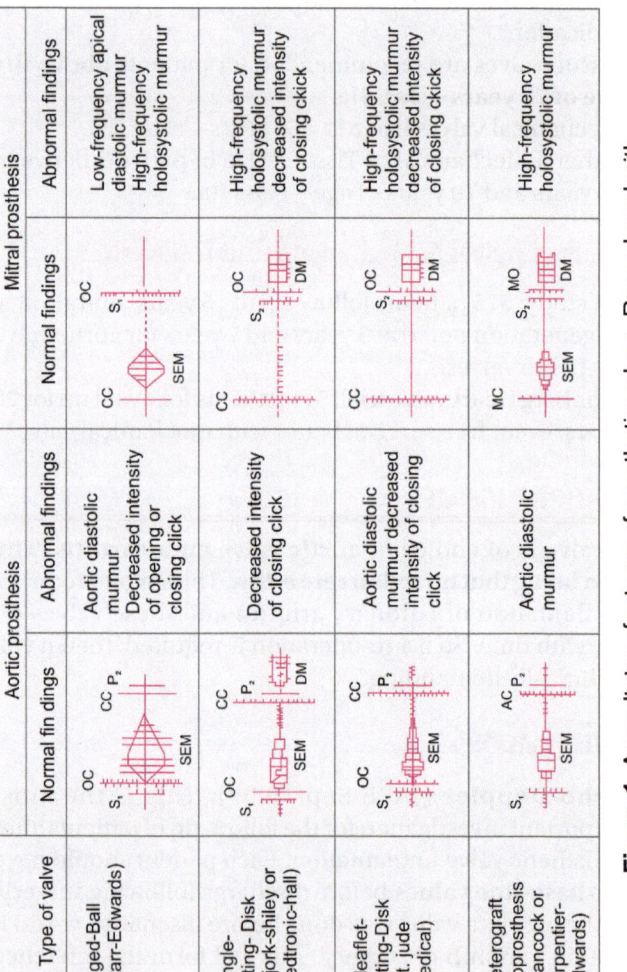

Figure 1 Auscultatory features of prosthetic valves. Reproduced with permission from Vongpatanasin et al. NEJM 1996[2]

Table 1
Doppler parameters for MVR

	Normal	Possible	Stenosis
Velocity m/sec	<1.9	1.9–2.5	>2.5
Mean	<5	6–10	>10
VTI ratio pros VTI/LVO	<2.2	2.2–2.5	>2.5
PHT	130	130–200	>200

Table 2
Doppler parameters for AVR

	Normal	Possible	Stenosis
Velocity m/sec	3	3-4	>4
Mean gradient	<20	20-35	35
DVI	0.30 or more	0.29 – 0.25	<0.25
EOA	>1.2	1.2 -0.8	<0.8
AT (ms)	<80	80 -100	>100

2. Fluroscopy - Cath Lab.: Diminished movement of the leaflet suggests thrombosis and excessive motion suggests that the base has come off due to separation
3. MRI: All the modern valves are MRI safe. It is usually done only when other imaging modalities are inconclusive.
4. Cardiac Cath: With the advent of Echo, this is rarely used to assess the valve gradients.

COMPLICATIONS

1. **Prosthetic valve thrombosis (PVT)**
    - **Incidence:** For MVR 0.35% and for AVR **0.1%** per year
    - **Clinical:** Sudden onset of severe breathlessness, pulmonary edema, cardiac arrest. Valve sounds are not heard well.
    - **Echo:** Gradient is increased across the valve; the valve opening is restricted.
    - **Fluroscopy:** The valve mobility is restricted.
    - **Treatment: Lysis or Surgery**
    - **Lysis: Lysis is given as short protocol or long protocol**. The latter is used if the patient is stable. If patient is **unstable then short protocol is used which is similar to STEMI protocol. The long protocols are given below: (Preferred one)**
        1. **Streptokinas**e: 500,000 units in 20 minutes, followed by 1.5 million **over 10 hours** without heparin is the commonly used regimen. OR

2. **rTpa** : 10 mg bolus, 50 mg over first hour, 20 mg second hour, 20 mg third hour OR **10 mg bolus followed by 90 mg over 9 hours** OR
3. **Tenecteplase** (JAPI 2012; 60: 55-60): This drug has been used at a dose of 1mg/kg as bolus in a group of 10 patients successfully.

- **Efficacy of Streptokinase Short versus Long Protocol**

  In a study done from AIIMS of Delhi, they found the overall efficacy of SK is only **59%**. This study also noted that there was not much difference between the short versus long protocol.[3]

2. **Surgery:** Patient is in class 3-4 **or** large clot burden (area more than 0.8 sq. cm).
3. **UFH: This is an alternative mode of treatment** for patients in class 1-2 and small clot burden. Small clot burden is defined as 5 mm of thrombus in most studies or as thrombus area less than 0.8 sq.cm.

Indications for Lysis or Surgery (ACC/AHA March 2014)
1. **Lysis is reasonable for patients with thrombosed left sided prosthetic valve of recent onset < 14 days, class 1 or 2 symptoms and a small thrombus of size < 0.8 sq.cm**
2. **Surgery is recommended for patients who are in class 3 or 4 or large thrombus of size > 0.8 sq cm**

Prognosis: Emergency surgery has a mortality of 15%. Lysis has a mortality of 10% with a risk of embolism of 15%.

2. Embolism

The common destination of the embolism is to the brain.
- **Incidence**: 4% per year if uncoagulated, 2% per year if on aspirin and 1% per year if on warfarin.
- **Risk factors**: Age > 70 years, mitral valve replacement, double valve replacement, ball and cage type of valve.
- **In all cases do a CT scan to exclude a bleed.**

3. Endocarditis (PVE)

Classification: Divided into early and late; early if it occurs within 60 days; late means if it occurs after 60 days. The reason for such a classification is that, the organisms causing endocarditis in the early phase is due to hospital acquired ones.

4. Valve Dysfunction

- **Stenosis:** This can happen either due to pannus formation or thrombus obstructing the valve. The gradients are increased and if the patient is symptomatic then immediate treatment is warranted.

- **Regurgitation:** This occurs secondary to infective endocarditis which results in paravalvular regurgitation. Mild central jets of regurgitation are common and they should not be mistaken as pathological.
- *Paravaular leak management*: It is due to suture dehiscence. The reasons are: 1. Infection, 2. Technical, 3. Heavily calcified valve 3.8% per year for mitral valve in one series. (EJE 2009) Usually surgery is done but nowadays it is being closed by device
- **Structural Valve Deterioration - SVD:** These tissue valves **deteriorate with time and also related to the patients age.** Given below is the relationship between age and valve failure at 10 years.

Age		Failure
Age < 40 years	–	40%
40–49 years	–	30%
50–59 years	–	20%
60–69 years	–	15%
70 years or more	–	10%

Porcine versus Pericardial Valve

- Carpentier Edwards Perimount valve has a more favorable rate of SVD than porcine valves.
- Structural Valve Degeneration – SVD: For porcine valves it starts at 7–8 years and for bovine pericardial valves at 11–12 years.[4]

5. Hemolysis

Hemolysis occurs when there is acute para valvular regurgitation. The Hemoglobin is low, reticulocytes are increased. Treatment consists replacing the valve. Nowadays, the paravalvular leak is closed with intracardiac devices.

■ EXCESSIVE ANTICOAGULATION – ACC/AHA GUIDELINES 2014

1. Excessive anticoagulation (INR greater than 5) greatly increases the risk of hemorrhage.
   Rapid decreases in INR below the therapeutic level increase the risk of thromboembolism.
2. **INR of 5 to 10 and not bleeding:** Withhold warfarin and monitor.
3. **INR more than 10 and not bleeding:** (a) Withhold Warfarin, (b) 1 to 2.5 mg of oral vitamin K1 (phytonadione). (c) The INR should be determined after 24 h and subsequently as needed. Warfarin therapy is restarted and adjusted dose appropriately to ensure that the INR is in the therapeutic range.
4. **In emergency situations:** (a) F**resh frozen plasma is preferable to high-dose vitamin** K1, (b) **Low-dose intravenous vitamin K (1 mg) appears safe in this**

situation. Yiu et al.[5] in a RCT of 102 patients compared IV vitamin K 1 mg versus FFP for patients with mechanical heart valves with INR values between 4-7. Six hours after treatment, patients in the FFP group had a significantly lower mean INR compared with the vitamin K group (2.75 ± 0.06 vs 3.44 ± 0.10, p = 0.01). No patient in both groups had over-correction (INR <2). One week later, there was no significant difference in mean INR between both groups (2.7 ± 0.11 vs 2.56 ± 0.12, p = 0.41). There were no adverse reactions or outcomes in both groups and they concluded that intravenous low-dose vitamin K is a safe alternative to FFP infusion for warfarin overdose in patients with mechanical prosthetic valves.

BRIDGING THERAPY[6] (TABLE 3)

This term is used when patients on warfarin for prosthetic valve need to discontinue the same for a procedure such as dental or surgery. During the time patient is off warfarin, either heparin or LMWH is given till the warfarin is re-introduced.

1. **AVR with no risk factors**: Warfarin be stopped 48 to 72 hours before the procedure (so the INR falls to less than 1.5) and restarted within 24 hours after the procedure. **Heparin is usually unnecessary**. On the day of surgery INR should be less than 1.5.
2. **MVR or AVR with risk factors:** Stop warfarin 3 days prior, overlap with heparin or LMWH and on the day of surgery restart as soon as bleeding stability allows.

Table 3
Bridging therapy – Summary

Day	To do	Comments
3 Day prior to surgery	Stop Warfarin	Check INR daily morning
Day 2 prior to surgery	LMWH: Fragmin/Clexane	If INR less than 2
Day 1 prior to surgery	Continue same LMWH	
Day of Surgery	No LMWH morning dose	INR should be less than 1.5 before surgery
	Start warfarin post-surgery at 6 pm	
	LMWH evening dose if no bleeding issues	
Postoperative Day 2	LMWH plus warfarin	
Postoperative Day 3	Warfarin only if INR more than 2	

3. **For emergency surgery:** Give **fresh frozen plasma** and proceed.
   Risk factors:
   - Atrial fibrillation
   - Previous thromboembolism
   - LV dysfunction
   - Hypercoagulable conditions
   - Older-generation thrombogenic valves
   - Mechanical tricuspid valve
   - Double valve replacement.

In one study that included 215 patients with mechanical valves, the risk of thromboembolism was 0.62%, using the above mentioned bridging therapy.

CORONARY ANGIOGRAM BEFORE VALVE SURGERY

1. Chest pain,
2. Objective evidence of ischemia
3. Known CAD
4. Risk factors for CAD
5. Decreased LV systolic function
6. Asymptomatic persons: Male above the age of 40 or post-menopausal women or other risk factors.

Coronary CT angio is an alternative to invasive coronary angio if the patient has no angina or LV dysfunction.

HEART FAILURE AFTER VALVE REPLACEMENT

Many patients after successful valve replacement come back with signs of heart failure. Some of the reasons are as follows:
1. Prosthetic valve stenosis or regurgitation – valve dysfunction.
2. Progression of another valve disease.
3. Pulmonary hypertension.
4. Tricuspid regurgitation – late onset.
5. Arrhythmia induced cardiomyopathy.

AFIB ABLATION DURING MITRAL VALVE REPLACEMENT

During MVR Atrial Fib ablation to restore to sinus rhythm has been attempted in many studies. In a recent RCT it was shown that at 1 year only 60% are in sinus rhythm and many patients needed pacemaker thereafter. (17%). [7]

TRANS CATHETER AORTIC VALVE REPLACEMENT[8] (TAVI OR TAVR)

Two types of prosthesis have now been approved. They are namely the Medtronic CoreValve and Edwards SAPIEN valve. In 2002, Cribier et al. did the first human implantation. The aortic valve is approached through the retrograde approach from the femoral artery or from left ventricle transapical approach. The following are the **criteria to accept a patient** for this procedure.

TAVR Indications (Vahanian et al.) – all 4 criteria need to be met.

1. Severe AS
2. Severe symptoms
3. Patients with contraindications for surgery
4. Life expectancy more than one year.

Contraindications

1. Size of the annulus varies from one type to another. < 18 mm or > 25 mm for SAPIEN valve
2. Bicuspid AV
3. Asymmetric calcification
4. Aortic root > 45
5. LV apical thrombus.

Complications[9]

1. Stroke: 3 to 4%
2. Paravalvular leak: 6–7%
3. Pacemaker: 13% versus 3% for SAVR
4. Vascular access complications
5. Thromboembolic complications.

Limitations between Medtronic and Edwards Sapien Valves (Circulation 2014;130:2321–2331)

Medtronic Corevalve	Edwards Sapien XT
Limits	Limits
Not repositionable	Not repositionable
Not retrievable	Not retrievable
Axial alignment of MCV depends on anatomy	Axial alignment of MCV depends on anatomy
High pacemaker rate	No anatomic implantation
Frame expands into ascending aorta partially covering the coronaries	Risk of annular rupture
Final movement in moment of release	Paravalvular leaks
Paravalvular leaks	Single shot procedure

REFERENCES

1. Emmert MY, et al. JACC interventions. 2011;822-3.
2. Vongpatanasin, et al. Prosthetic heart valves. NEJM. 1996;335:407-16.

3. Karthikkeyan, et al. Circulation. 2009;120:1108-14.
4. Huang G, Rahimtoola. Prosthetic Heart valve. Circulation. 2011;123:2602-5.
5. Yiu, et al. American Journal of Cardiology. 2006;97:409-11.
6. Bonow et al. Guidelines for valvular heart disease JACC; 2008;e1-e142.
7. Gillinov et al. Surgical ablation of atrial fibrillation during mitral valve surgery. NEJM. 2015.
8. Percutaneous aortic valve therapy. Heart. 2009;95:1538-46.
9. Falk V, Circulation 2014;130:2332-42.

CHAPTER 19

Hypertrophic Cardiomyopathy

Jacob Jose

CHAPTER OUTLINE

- Prevalence
- Pathogenesis
- Genes Associated with HCM
- Family Screening
- Clinical Features
- ECG
- ECHO
- Electrophysiologic Studies
- Hemodynamics
- Sudden Death
- Natural History
- Drug Therapy
- Surgery
- Alcohol Septal Ablation

DEFINITION

In an adult, hypertrophic cardiomyopathy (HCM) is defined by a **wall thickness ≥15 mm** in one or more LV myocardial segments—as measured by any imaging technique.

PREVALENCE

The overall prevalence is estimated to be **1 in 500.** On ECG screening the prevalence is estimated to be 0.2% and 5% by Echocardiographic screening of the population.

PATHOGENESIS

1. Abnormal calcium metabolism: Increased calcium flux in the sarco reticulum is associated with abnormal and asymmetric growth.
2. Abnormal penetrating coronary arteries producing focal ischemia.
3. Abnormal adrenergic stimulation of the heart.

The anatomical and functional features of obstructive HCM include:

1. A narrow **LVOT** diameter: An LVOT diameter of 20 mm or less is associated with obstruction in 66% of patients.[1]
2. Increased velocity of blood flow producing a **venturi** effect.

3. Anterior and central displacement of the **papillary muscles** with typically elongated chordae.
4. The **mitral leaflets** are longer, the annulus to coaptation point is more distal and the **coaptation point is in the body of the leaflets** (Mean 9 mm from the anterior leaflet tip versus within 3 mm of the leaflet tip). The elongation of the leaflet can be for the anterior leaflet or the middle of the posterior leaflet. In a small group the **anterolateral papillary muscle may insert** directly into the leaflet without the chordae which may produce mid-cavity obstruction.

Myocardial Fibrosis

Myocardial fibrosis is a hallmark of hypertrophic cardiomyopathy and a proposed substrate for arrhythmias and heart failure. In animal models, profibrotic genetic pathways are activated early, before hypertrophic remodeling. A study was done in 39 subjects showed that there were elevated levels of Procollagen C-peptide in the serum. This profibrotic state preceded the development of left ventricular hypertrophy or fibrosis visible on MRI.[2]

Types of Asymmetric Hypertrophy

1. Septal
2. Apical
3. Mid-ventricular.

Causes of Myocardial Ischemia

1. Increased demand due to hypertrophy.
2. Decreased capillary density.
3. Reduced vasodilatory reserve.
4. Systolic compression.
5. Abnormal intramural coronary arteries.

Mitral Regurgitation in HCM

Eject obstruct-leak: During the middle of systole, there is anterior and basal movement of AML, resulting in **failure of coaptation,** which is responsible for mitral regurgitation.

GENES ASSOCIATED WITH HCM

In the last 25 years of research has now identified nearly 11 genes with more than 1400 mutations. An excellent review is published.[3] Table 1 and Figure 1 gives the prevalence of various genetic abnormalities observed.

Table 1
Mutations in genes for cardiac sarcomeric proteins causally linked to HCM

Sarcomeric protein	Chromosome	Prevalence
β-Myosin heavy chain	14	35%
Cardiac troponin T	1	15%
α–Tropomyosin	15	5%
Cardiac Troponin I	19	25%
Myosin Light Chains	3,12	25%
With WPW	7	5%
Myosin Binding Protein C	11	15%

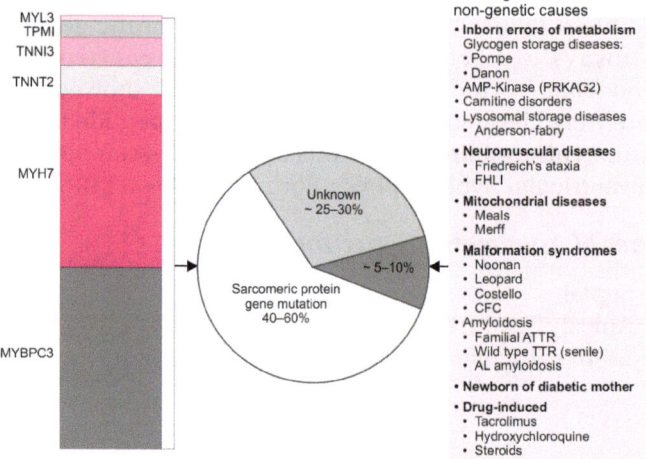

Figure 1 Genetic and non-genetic causes of HCM.
Source: Adapted from Task Force of ESC guidelines Sept 2014

FAMILY SCREENING BY ECHO OR CMR [4] (JACC JULY 2012)

1. Below 12 years findings are rare; screening if malignant family history or competitive sports.
2. 12–21 years: Echo every 12 to 18 months.
3. 22 years or more: Every 5 years.

CLINICAL FEATURES—OBSTRUCTIVE CARDIOMYOPATHY (FIG. 2)

1. **Dyspnea:** The most common symptom - 90%
2. **Angina** is present in 75% of cases. Many patients with HCM experience postprandial exacerbation of their symptoms. The vasodilation associated with eating may be deleterious in HCM especially during exercise (JACC 1991;18:429-36).

3. **Syncope: Causes**: (Circulation editorial. 2009;119: 1697-99). (a) Arrhythmia: Paroxysmal AFib, Complete heart block or sustained VT, (b) Hemodynamic: LVOT obstruction Symptoms of impaired consciousness (syncope and pre-syncope) occur in ~15-25% of the patients with HCM. In young patients, a history of recurrent syncope is associated with an increased risk of sudden death. Syncope typically occurs in younger patients with smaller ventricles. Impaired consciousness is often provoked by **exercise (either during or after) or by postural change**. However, episodes can occur at rest and are often worse post-prandially. Syncope usually occurs without warning and/or symptoms suggestive of the cause. It is said to be more common in patients with resting LV outflow tract gradients.
4. **Reversed pulsus paradoxus**: An inspiratory increase in arterial pressure (reversed pulsus paradoxus) can be seen in these patients. During inspiration, the negative intrathoracic pressure leads to a higher transmural aortic pressure and increased afterload. This in turn leads to a reduction in the severity of dynamic obstruction and an increase in LV stroke volume and, therefore, arterial pressure.
5. **JVP:** Prominent A wave; the mean pressure is normal.
6. **Carotid pulse**: Rapid and jerky.
7. **Apical impulse**: Spike and dome.
5. **S4**
6. S3
7. **Second sound** is paradoxical by split in severe cases.
8. **Systolic murmur**, crescendo–decrescendo radiation to base and to apex. Systolic murmur is best heard at the third and fourth intercostal spaces. The murmur is crescendo–decrescendo.
9. **Mitral regurgitant murmur.**
10. **Mitral leaflet**: Septal contact sound.
11. **Aortic regurgitant murmur.**
12. **Mid diastolic murmur** at apex.
13. **Ejection sound from Aorta.**

Mid-Ventricular Obstruction

1. Apical systolic murmur 2/6 or 3/6.
2. Long mitral diastolic murmur due to mid-ventricular. obstruction and asynchronous relaxation.
3. Bifid pulse or double apex or Mitral leaflet septal contact sound are never found.
4. Paradoxical split may be present

2 systolic marmur; 2 diastolic murmur; 2 systolic sounds

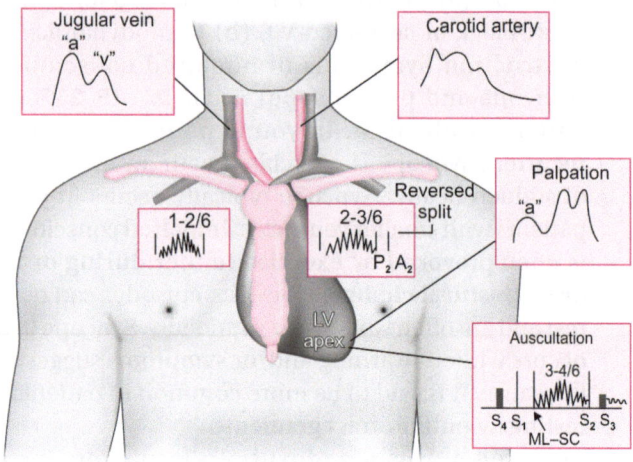

Figure 2 Auscultatory features of HCM

Valsalva and HCM

This method was first used to expel pus from the ear in the year 1704. Forced expiration against closed glottis for 10 seconds OR you can ask the patient to blow into a mercury manometer to keep the pressure to 40 mmHg for 10 seconds.

Effect of Valsalva in HCM Murmur

Valsalva Strain—Murmur Increases
Valsalva Release—Murmur Decreases.

Identification of the Phases of the Valsalva

In phase 2, there is an increase of pulse rate; In phase 4, there is reflex bradycardia.

Alcohol and Obstructive HCM[5]

Alcohol consumed socially in one cocktail can cause 63% increase in LVOT gradient.

Table 2

Methods to differentiate obstructive vs nonobstructive HCM

	Obstructive	Non-obstructive
JVP A wave	Prominent	Prominent
Carotid pulse	Jerky	Normal
Palpable S4	Common	Common
Systolic thrill	Present	Not present
Triple ripple	Present	Not present
Murmur	Long, louder	Shorter or absent

Yamaguchi's Apical HCM

1. Apical motion may be dyskinetic.
2. Giant T inversion in ECG.
3. Spade-shaped LV cavity in angiography
4. MR is rare.
5. Seen in Japan.
6. Echo - IVRF flow is directed away from the apex.
7. It is not genetically determined. Not associated with severe symptoms. Risk factors for sudden death are not there.
8. 3–10% of all cases of HCM.
9. Two complications are peculiar to Apical CMY. Apical ischemia followed by apical infarction will lead on to mid-cavity obstruction. This may give rise to ventricular arrhythmias. Atrial Fib is more common with elevated filling pressure.

ECG FEATURES OF HCM

1. ST – T changes
2. LVH
3. Giant T wave inversions
4. Prominent q waves: inferior leads or Precordial leads
5. Left axis deviation
6. LAE
7. Pre-excitation
8. In **only 6% of cases the ECG is likely to be normal.**

ECHO

1. Left Ventricular Hypertrophy

The left ventricular hypertrophy is the hallmark of HCM. Two scoring systems have been in use and they are given below:

Wiggle's scoring:

- Basal   15 – 19   1
                20 – 24   2
                25-30   3
                > 30   4
- Basal 2/3rds   2
- Apex   2
- Anterolateral   2
  Total   **10**

Maron's classification:

Type 1	– 10%	Anterior septum
Type 2	– 20%	Anterior and inferior septum
Type 3	– 52%	Anterior + Inferior + lateral septum
Type 4		other than septum

2. M – mode Echo features of obstruction: SAM and Aortic valve notch

1. Systolic anterior motion of AML (SAM) **Grading of SAM**: Gilbert et al
   - 0 absent
   - 1. mild; minimal mitral-septal distance >10 mm during systole
   - 2. moderate; minimal mitral-septal distance ≤10 mm during systole
   - 3. marked; brief or prolonged contact between the AMVL and septum.[6]

   The severity of SAM can be inferred from the **duration** of leaflet/chordal contact with the septum, being mild if contact occurs for <10% of systole, and **severe if >30% of systole**.[7]

2. Aortic valve notch in M mode indicates LVOT obstruction.

3. LVOT gradient

- Echo LVOT gradient is 15 to 25 mm Hg **greater than** that obtained in the cath lab due to pressure recovery phenomenon.
- The **jet is dagger shaped** and looks like a lobster because of the mid-systolic drop in the gradient.[8] This mid-systolic velocity drop (MSD) occurs in patients with gradients above 60 mmHg.[9]
- The LVOT jet of HCM may be confused with MR jet that often co-exists (Table 3).

4. Left atrial enlargement

LA diameter more than 40 mm or area > 20 cm^2 is frequently seen in the four chamber view and this is due to diastolic dysfunction and mitral regurgitation.

False positive diagnosis of HCM in Echo or misdiagnosis of HCM

1. RV papillary muscle and prominent trabeculations that overlie the ventricular septum

Table 3

Methods to differentiate LVOT jet vs mitral regurgitation jet

	LVOT jet	Mitral regurgitation jet
Onset	Aortic valve opening	Initiation of systole
Duration	Left ventricular ejection	Holosystolic
Peak velocity usually	<4.5 m/sec	>4.5 m/sec
Contour	Dagger-shaped	Symmetrical
Timing of peak velocity	Delayed	Early systole

2. LV pseudo tendon.
3. Sigmoid septum.
4. Athletic heart.
5. ASH in the presence of Aortic stenosis or HTN.

ELECTROPHYSIOLOGIC STUDIES

1. Abnormal in 80%.
2. Sinus Node Dysfunction in 66%.
3. HV interval abnormalities in 30%.
4. Ability to induce VT in 43%.
5. Accessory pathway in 5%.

HEMODYNAMICS

1. **Post VPC accentuation of gradient:**
   There is increase in contractility in the beat following the extrasystole that it **outweighs** the otherwise salutary effect of increased volume caused by the compensatory pause and produces an increase in gradient and often the murmur as well (**Brokenbrough Braunwald Morrow sign** - Augmented LV pressure with concomitant decrease in the aortic systolic and pulse pressure). In some patients the post-extrasystolic murmur is attenuated despite an increase in the outflow gradient apparently in this setting the murmur is mirroring to a greater degree changes in the severity of mitral regurgitation rather than changes in the outflow gradient.
2. **Isoprin infusion:** Isoprin infusion increases the gradient by increasing the contractility.

NATURAL HISTORY

- 20 years murmur detected.
- 30 years NYHA 2.
- 35 years class 3.
- 40 years class 4 or death.

Annual mortality is 3% per year, in younger individuals it may be 6% per year

SUDDEN DEATH

Risk factors for sudden death (Adapted from ESC guidelines 2006)
Major Risk Factors (7 of them have been listed).
1. Cardiac arrest (Ventricular fibrillation).
2. Spontaneous sustained ventricular tachycardia.
3. Family history of sudden death (one or more first degree relative younger than 40 years of age).

4. **Syncope** (**Two or more episodes syncope within one year – some text say 6 months**) An article that was published in Circulation April 2009 based on 1511 consecutive patients with HCM, patients with unexplained syncope less than 6 months had a 5 fold risk. Also, patients over the age of 40 years and more than 5 years ago, did not have higher risk.[10]
5. **Holter**: NSVT (one or more runs are with a rate higher than 120 beats per minute and duration of less than 30 seconds.
6. **Treadmill Testing:** Abnormal blood pressure response to exercise. Failure to increase the blood pressure to 25 mm Hg, during exercise or if there is a fall in BP of more than 10 mmHg with exercise.[11]
7. **Echo**: LVH – more than 30 mm.[12]

SCD Risk Modifiers

This is a term introduced in the ACC/AHA guidelines of 2011. These are to be used for AICD consideration when the risk remains borderline after taking into account the conventional risk factors.
1. **CMR – LGE > 15%.**
2. LV apical aneurysm (10% annual event rate).
3. Gene - Double or compound mutations.
4. Marked LVOT obstruction defined as 30 mm of Hg or more.

Gene Mutations and Survival

- Arginine mutations are associated with premature death before 35 years.

SCD Risk Calculation Formula (ESC Aug 2014 Guidelines)[13] (Figure 3)

This calculator is available online and it involves the following variables:
1. Age at clinical evaluation.
2. LV maximal wall thickness.
3. LA diameter.
4. Family history of SCD.
5. Syncope.
6. LVOT gradient.
7. NSVT.

ESC Guidelines for ICD Implantation - 2014

Score is calculated using multiple variables and based on risk ICD is recommended.

Chapter 19: Hypertrophic Cardiomyopathy

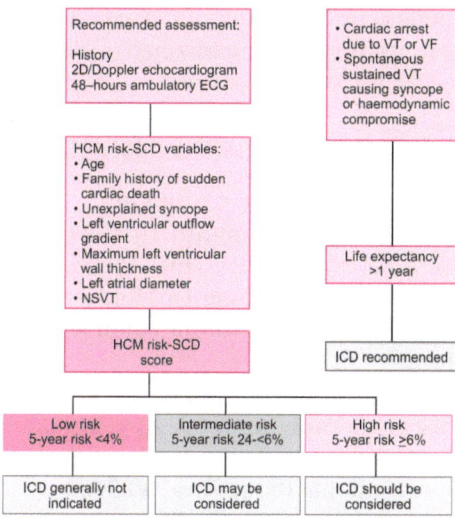

Figure 3 SCD calculator ESC

TMT Testing in HCM

- It is a class 2a indication.
- Useful in 3 situations: 1. To identify latent obstruction, 2. Rule out CAD and 3. High risk.
- For SCD risk – negative predictive value is higher and if abnormal we will need further stratification.

TREATMENT

1. Drug therapy: Beta blocker/Verapamil/Disopyramide.
2. SCD risk stratification for all and then decide on ICD.
3. PTSMA; Alcohol septal ablation.
4. Surgery: Septal Myectomy – Morrow procedure with or without correction of mitral valve apparatus.

DRUG THERAPY

1. Beta blockers are generally the **initial choice** for patients with symptomatic HCM and/or effective in 60–80% of patients.
2. Verapamil is given for patients **who cannot tolerate beta blockers**. Death has been reported in patients with severe symptoms, pulmonary hypertension and severe outflow tract infection. Hence verapamil should not be used in these groups of patients.
3. For patients who are not controlled with the beta blocker addition of **Disopyramide** should be considered since its negative inotropic effect further decreases the gradient. It is recommended that Disopyramide be given with a beta blocker to prevent a rapid ventricular response if atrial

fibrillation occurs. In a study of 118 patients followed for 3 years or more, 66% were maintained on this drug without the need for further procedures.[14]

SURGERY—MYECTOMY/MORROW PROCEDURE

- **Is the preferred primary treatment**
- Dr Cleland of Hammersmith Hospital was the first surgeon to do myectomy.[15] This was abandoned in UK for several decades and later Dr Morrow of NIH, Kirklin in Mayo and Williams of Toronto pioneered the surgical procedure.
- Sudden death is not eliminated by surgery but the incidence is certainly reduced. 10-year follow up study of patients with obstructive cardiomyopathy following surgery suggest that the survival is 83%.[16]
- Surgical mortality is < 5% overall, but mortality in patients younger than 40 is 1%.
- Nowadays resection of IVS is combined with mitral valve correction as well. The procedure selection is as follows[17]:
  – IVS less than 18 mm and AML > 30 mm: Resection of IVS minimal, Plicate the AML, Release the Papillary muscle.
  – IVS > 18 mm and AML > 30 mm: Resect IVS + Plicate AML + Release papillary muscle.
  – !VS > 18 mm and AML < 30 mm: Resect the IVS + Release the papillary muscle.

ALCOHOL SEPTAL ABLATION (PTSMA)[18]

In 1995, D. Ulrich Sigwart injected a small quantity alcohol absolute alcohol into the first septal artery of a 67-year-old woman with HCM and hence, this procedure is called as **Sigwart** procedure. Also called as **PTSMA**; Percutaneous Transluminal Septal Myocardial Ablation; also called as **TASH** – **T**rans coronary **A**blation of **S**eptal **H**ypertrophy.

Effects of PTSMA on the Conduction System

New RBBB developed in 46% of patients and first degree AV block in 53% of patients.

The need for permanent pacemaker is higher in:
1. Females.
2. More than one septal artery is treated.
3. Pre-exciting LBBB. PTSMA causes transmural infarction in the basal mid-septum close to involving right bundle.

Predictors for Complete Heart Block

Complete AV block is a serious complication of PTSMA. This can happen during the procedure or after several

days later. Intraprocedural complete heart block can occur in **20%** of patients. In a study done in 172 patients, showed that the following **factors** could predict the need for pacemaker.[19]
1. **QRS duration > 120 msec before or after (LBBB).**
2. **First degree AV block.**
3. Retrograde AV block on EP.
4. Age > 58 years.
5. Female.

Patients who developed retrograde AV block and one other risk factor had a 26% risk of complete AV block.

Complications of PTSMA

- Early mortality of 30 days is 1.5% and late mortality 0.5%.
- LAD dissection 1.8%.
- Pericardial effusion 0.6%.
- Complete AV block –See above.

PTSMA Concerns

1. Risk of long-term arrhythmias: The scar that is created, is likely to cause arrhythmias.
2. PTSMA is recommended and done much more early than surgery. The concern is that, whether they are all indicated. This procedure can be justified only if the patient is symptomatic.

Indications

Symptomatic NYHA 3 or 4 despite drug therapy with resting or provocable peak gradient of 50 mmHg or more with septal thickness more than 18 mm.

Technique

- Which wire? – Any floppy wire
- Which guiding cath? JL or XB – LAD
- Which balloon? – Over the wire
- How to select the septal artery? Inject any echo contrast to see how much of the septum is visualized.
- How do you confirm that the balloon has been positioned properly? Inject the contrast through the balloon to see that contrast does not reflux back to the LAD
- How much Alcohol? – We inject 0.3 ml per injection to a maximum of 4 injections.
- **What is a success?** A reduction of gradient to 30 mmHg or > 50% reduction of provocable gradient.

Survival—Long Term Results for PTSMA

In the North American Registry data of 874 patients the survival at 1, 5 and 9 years were 97%, 86% and 74% respectively.[20]

Radiofrequency Septal Ablation for HCM

There has been interest in the use of Radiofrequency for ablation for HCM. This has been tried out in both adults and children.[21] In a study of 32 children at a median age of 11 years, using cool tip ablation catheter via a femoral approach was found to be useful with one death and one patient needing pacemaker.

PTSMA versus Surgical Myectomy

There are major anatomical differences between these two procedures are well made out by MRI and they are summarized in the Table 4:[22]

Table 4
Anatomical differences of PTSMA versus Myectomy

	PTSMA	Myectomy
Site	Inferior part of the septum extending onto right ventricle	LV side of the septum both basal and middle
Depth	Transmural in basal septum, non-transmural in midventricular septum	10 mm in depth
Mass resection	16 ± 9 gm	6 ± 4 gm
Resection of basal septum	Spared in 25%	All patients

PTSMA versus Myectomy—Survival Differences

It has been hotly debated whether survival following PTSMA is as good as Surgery. In a retrospective analysis from Mayo clinic data base of 177 patients it was found that 8-year survival estimate was 79% versus 79%; thus long-term survival was favorable and similar for surgery and PTSMA.[23]

DIFFERENTIAL DIAGNOSIS OF HCM

There are several conditions that can look like HCM on the imaging such as Athletic heart and conditions such as Danon's disease. They are summarized in Tables 5 and 6.

- LV **wall thickness of > 13 mm together with LA size of 41 mm** should effectively rule out the diagnosis of athletes' heart.

Table 5
Differential diagnosis from atheletic heart

	HCM	Athletic heart
LV wall thickness	More than 16 in males and 14 in females	Less than 15 mm
LVIDD	Less than 45 mm	>55 mm
LA	>41 mm	<40
LV filling e' less than 9 Or E/e' >15	Abnormal	Normal
SAM and gradient	Present	No
Family history	Possible	No
Regression of wall thickness with detraining for 3 months	No	Possible

- Some experts feel that LV cavity size in diastole of **45 mm or less is the single most** important discriminator for HCM than Athletic heart. [24]

Table 6
Differential diagnosis of thick ventricular walls (JACC April 27, 2010)

Condition	Age at presentation	Clinical	Echo
Mucopoly-saccharidosis	1–20 years Median 10 years		
Fabrys	Male 11 years Female 23 years	Neuropathic pain	Normal EF Symmetrical LVH
Danon	<20 years	Heart failure skeletal myopathy mental retardation	LV very thick 20–60 mm
Friedreich ataxia	<25 years	Gait	
Cardiac oxalosis	>20 years	Renal stones	Symmetrical LVH
HCM	17 to 18 years	Dyspnea/Angina	Asymmetrical LVH
Hypertensive heart disease	>30 years	History of HTN	Concentric LVH

- **2% of athletes** approximately develop Athletic heart.
- It takes **two years** of intensive training of at least five hours per week to induce these adaptive changes.
- Athletic heart is common with **endurance training** when compared to those involved in strength training.
- Athletic LVH primarily increased septal thickness, females up to 13 mm, and males up to 16 mm.

HCM and Pregnancy

- Maternal mortality is uncommon, because though there is a decrease in the afterload which should exacerbate the LVOT gradient, this is offset by the increase in the maternal increase in the plasma volume.
- The main risk is for the fetus – 50% chance of occurrence for HCM.
- Some patients may need a small dose of diuretics

REFERENCES

1. Pollick C, Rakowski H, Wigle ED. Muscular subaortic stenosis; the quantitative relationship between systolic anterior motion and the pressure gradient. Circulation. 1984;69:43-7.
2. Carolyn, et al. Myocardial fibrosis as an early manifestation of hypertrophic cardiomyopathy. NEJM. 2010;363:552-63.
3. Maron BJ, Maron J, Semsarian C. Genetics of Hypertrophic cardiomyopathy. JACC 2012;60:705-15.
4. Ho CY, Seidman. Contemporary approach to hypertrophic cardiomyopathy. Circulation. 2006;113:e858-e62.
5. Rami Paz, et al. The effect of the ingestion of ethanol on obstruction of the left ventricular outflow tract in hypertrophic cardiomyopathy. NEJM. 1996;335:938-41.
6. Gilbert BW, Pollick C, Adelman AG, Wigle ED: Hypertrophic cardiomyopathy: sub classification by M-mode echocardiography. Am J Cardiol. 1980:45:861.
7. Williams. Echocardiography in Hypertrophic cardiomyopathy. European Journal of Echo. 2009:10:iii9.
8. Sherrid etl; Mid systolic drop in left ventricular velocity in obstructive hypertrophic cardiomyopathy; JASE.1997;10:707-12.
9. Barac I, et al. Effect of obstruction on longitudinal left ventricular modeling in hypertrophic cardiomyopathy; JACC. 2007;49:1203-11.
10. Spirito, et al. Syncope and HCM. Circulation. 2009;119:1703-10.
11. Matsumura Y, Elliott PM, Virdee MS, Sorajja P, Doi P, McKenna WJ. Left ventricular diastolic function assessed using Doppler tissue imaging in patients with hypertrophic cardiomyopathy: relation to symptoms and exercise capacity. Heart. 2002;87:247-51.

12. Spirito P, et al. Magnitude of left ventricular hypertrophy and risk of sudden death in hypertrophic cardiomyopathy. NEJM. 2000;342:1778-85.
13. ESC guidelines, EHJ Aug 2014, http://dx.doi.org/10.1093/eurheartj/ehu284
14. Sherrid MV, et al. Multicenter study of the efficacy and safety in obstructive hypertrophic cardiomyopathy. JACC. 2005;45:1251-8.
15. Cleland WP. The surgical management of obstructive cardiomyopathy. J Cardiovasc Surgery. 1963;4:489-91.
16. Ommen SR, et al. Long-term effects of surgical septal myectomy on survival in patients with obstructive hypertrophic cardiomyopathy. JACC. 2005;46:470-6.
17. Sherrid MV, et al. The mitral valve in obstructive cardiomyopathy. JACC. 2016;1846-58.
18. Faber L, Meissner A, Ziemssen P, Seggewiss H. Percutaneous transluminal septal myocardial ablation for hypertrophic obstructive cardiomyopathy: long term follow up of the first series of 25 patients. Heart 2000;83:326-31.
19. Thorsten, et al. Predictors of complete heart block after trans coronary ablation of septal hypertrophy. JACC. 2007;49:2356-63.
20. Nagueh et al. Alcohol septal ablation for the treatment of Hypertrophic cardiomyopathy. JACC. 2011;58:2322-8.
21. Narayanswamy Sreeram, et al. Radiofrequency septal reduction in hypertrophic cardiomyopathy in children, JACC. 2011;58:2501-10.
22. Veleti, et al. Comparison of surgical septal myectomy and alcohol septal ablation with cardiac magnetic resonance imaging in patients with hypertrophic obstructive cardiomyopathy. J Am Coll Cardiol. 2007;49:350-7.
23. Sorajja P, et al. Survival after alcohol septal ablation for hypertrophic cardiomyopathy, Circulation. 2012;126:2374-80.
24. Rawlins, et al. Left ventricular hypertrophy in athletes. European J Echocardiography. 2009;10:350-6.

Constrictive Pericorditis

Jacob Jose

CHAPTER OUTLINE

- Constrictive Pericarditis
- Hemodynamic Criteria

Patient with heart failure signs, such as elevated jugular venous pressure, ascites and pedal edema. The differential diagnosis includes the following:
- Constrictive pericarditis
- Restrictive cardiomyopathy, such as endomyocardial fibrosis or amyloidosis
- Tricuspid valve disease, such as organic TR secondary to Rheumatic or infective endocarditis
- Pulmonary hypertension with right heart failure
- Dilated cardiomyopathy with CCF
- Hypertrophic cardiomyopathy in late stages.

CONSTRICTIVE PERICARDITIS

Syndromes of Constrictive Pericarditis

- Chronic CP
- Subacute CP: weeks to months after pericarditis
- Postoperative CP
- Occult CP
- Localized CP
- Transient acute constriction
- Effusive constrictive pericarditis: Safrista–Saulda et al. defined this as **failure of RA pressure to decline** by at least 50% to a level below 10 mm Hg when pericardial pressure was reduced to near 0 mm Hg by pericardiocentesis.

Pathoanatomical Forms (ESC guidelines 2004;24:587-610)

- Annular form along the AV groove
- Left-sided
- Right-sided
- Global form
- Global form with myocardial atrophy
- Global form with myocardial fibrosis.

Etiology

- **Tuberculosis** can be the cause in 38–83% of cases (IHJ 2003;55:305-9)
- **Idiopathic is the most common cause worldwide**
- **In 18% of cases, the pericardium is not thickened** (Mayo clinic series).

Pathophysiology

- Failure of transmission of intrathoracic pressure changes during respiration to the cardiac chambers is an important contributor to the pathophysiology
- **During inspiration,** the decrease in left ventricular filling results in **leftward shift of septum allowing augmented flow into the right ventricle.**
  - With inspiration, the drop in intrathoracic pressure results in a decrease in pulmonary venous pressure. However the LV pressure does not fall since the drop in intrathoracic pressure is not transmitted to the LV
  - On inspiration, **the pulmonary vein to LA gradient is reduced**, and so the transmitral flow is reduced
  - So the LV becomes small and the septum shift, to the left and RV becomes bigger.

Clinical Signs of Constrictive Pericarditis

- JVP is elevated
- Friedrich's sign—Rapid Y descent
- Kussmauls—Inspiratory increase in venous pressure or failure to decrease on inspiration
- Pericardial Knock
- Paradoxical pulse is noted in one third of patients
- Tricuspid regurgitation murmur
- Wide split second heart sound
- Hepatomegaly
- Ascites out of proportion to the pedal edema (**ascites precox**—due to high RA pressure).

ECG Changes

- Left atrial enlargement (LAE)
- Low voltage
- Atrial Fib in one third of cases
- Nonspecific T wave changes.

Chest X-ray

- Cardiac size is normal to increased (increased if there is associated pericardial effusion
- Pericardial calcification is better seen by fluoroscopy

- Pleural effusion
- Pulmonary venous hypertension, if left filling pressures are elevated.

Echo Signs (Circulation Imaging May 2014)

- Septal bounce (sensitivity 93%, specificity 69%)
- Mitral inflow variation of more than 25% variation
- Mitral e' >9 cm/sec (sensitivity 83%, specificity 81%)
- E' ratio of medial to lateral >0.91
- Hepatic vein–expiratory diastolic reversal ratio >0.79
- TEE pericardial thickness is better made out
- Strain: Longitudinal strain preserved in basal and mid-segments with derangement in apical region. Circumferential strain is reduced (JASE Jan 2009).

An algorithm has been suggested by the ASE for the differentiating between constriction versus restriction (JASE April 2016). This utilizes five steps (Flowchart 1).

1. Mitral inflow E/A ratio more than 0.8 with dilated IVC as the first step.
2. Look at the ventricular septal motion.
3. Medial tissue Doppler e'.
4. Lateral e' less than medial e'.
5. Hepatic vein expiratory reversal.

Flowchart 1: Algorithm by ASE to differentiate between constriction versus restriction

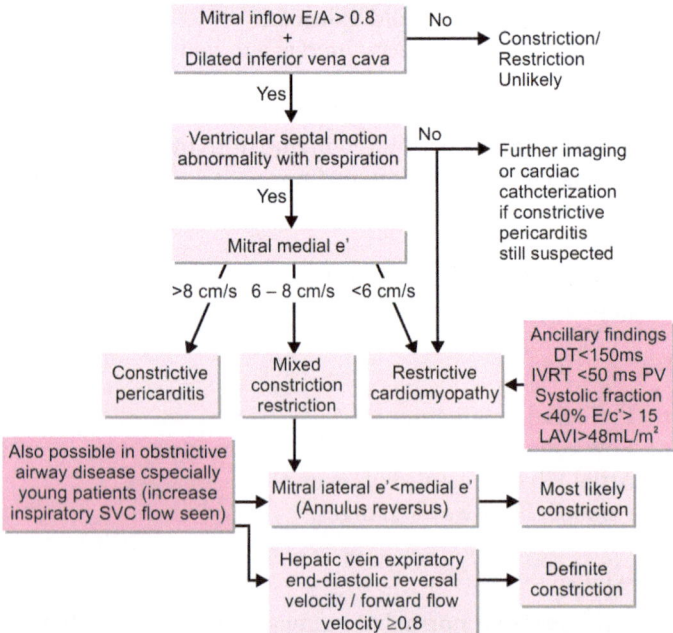

Source: ASE guidelines for diastolic dysfunction; JASE April 2016

HEMODYNAMIC CRITERIA

Criteria	Sensitivity (%)	Specificity (%)	PPV (%)	NPV (%)
Traditional LVEDP-RVEDP <5 mm Hg	60	38	4	57
RVEDP/RVSP >1/3	93	38	52	89
PASP <55 mm Hg	93	24	47	25
LV RFW ≥7 mm Hg	93	57	61	92
Respiratory change in RAP <3 mm Hg	93	48	58	92
Dynamic Respiratory PCWP/ LV respiratory gradient ≥5 mm Hg	93	81	78	94
LV/RV interdependence	100	95	94	100

Role of Cardiac MRI (JACC Oct 3rd, 2009)

- **Pericardial thickness**: Normal pericardial thickness is 2 mm or less. On Blood pool anatomical CMR, **more than 4 mm** thickness is considered abnormal
- **Cine MR**: Increased ventricular coupling with inspiratory flattening of the septum. This can be quantified in the short axis images in expiration versus inspiration. If the septal excursion is more than **12% it is very specific for CP**
- **Tagged cine MR**: Nonadherence of visceral and parietal pericardium throughout the cardiac cycle.

Pericardectomy

- Hospital mortality is around 5–15%. In CMC series the mortality was 11% (Thorax Aug 1988;637–641). In a series from AIIMS, the mortality was 7.6% (Annals of Thoracic Surgery. 2006;81:522–530)
- In only 60% of cases the hemodynamics will become normalized.

CHAPTER 21

Aortoarteritis

Ashish Kumar, Jacob Jose

CHAPTER OUTLINE

- Historical Perspective
- Etiopathogenesis
- Classification
- Clinical Features
- Criteria for Diagnosis
- Modified Diagnostic Criteria
- Natural History
- Uyama and Asayama Classification of Retinopathy
- Assessment of Disease Activity
- Investigations
- Treatment
- Medical Treatment
- Indications for Revascularization
- Coarctation of Aorta

DEFINITION

Takayasu's arteritis is a chronic inflammatory disease involving the aorta and its major branches and frequently the pulmonary arteries.

HISTORICAL PERSPECTIVE

The first mention of the disease is in 1856 by Savory and Kussmall. Takayasu is credited with describing the ocular manifestations of the disease in 1908 and Shimizu and Sano detailed the clinical features of the disease in 1948. The term Takayasu's arteritis came into existence in 1954.

ETIOPATHOGENESIS

The exact aetiology is not yet established. The proposed mechanisms are as follows:

1. *Autoimmune:* This is supported by finding of high gamma-globulins and circulating immune complexes (antiaorta antibodies and antiendothelial antibodies).
2. *Genetic susceptibility:* Supported by HLA associations. There is increased expression of B-5, B-21, BW52 and DR12. The expression of A-19, B-35, B-40 in Takayasu's arteritis is less.

Other proposed etiological factors like tuberculous infection and infestation by an unidentified nematode with arterial tropism have gone out of favor. The finding of an increase in CD4+: CD8+ ratio, a high basal protein kinase activity and a high intracellular calcium concentration reflect the activated state of circulating lymphocytes, but the stimulus for activation remains obscure. The infiltrating lymphocytes, especially the killer cells release a cytolytic factor called perforin, which plays a critical role in the vascular injury of Takayasu's arteritis.

Pathologically, Takayasu's arteritis is a panarteritis. The disease passes through the following phases:

1. *Inflammatory phase:* Granulomatous arteritis with secondary alterations in the media and adventitia with round cell infiltration.
2. *Sclerotic phase:* Intimal hyperplasia, medial degeneration and adventitial fibrosis.
3. *Obliterative phase:* Total disappearance of elastic lamina with obliteration of vasavasorum and arterial lumen.

In advanced cases, the aortic intima may have a tree-bark appearance similar to that of luetic aortitis. *Skipped areas of involvement is quite characteristic.* Even though the lumen may be critically narrowed, the outer diameter of the vessel is not significantly affected. The changes are most marked usually at the branch points of the arteries and the involvement of the left side is noted to be the more severe in case of involvement of either side.

The lesions are:
- Stenotic—85%
- Dilatative—2%
- Mixed—13%
- Aneurysms are seen in 2–26.7% cases. The aneurysmal form is more commonly associated with aortic regurgitation, elevated ESR and systemic hypertension. Aneurysms are generally considered a **late** manifestation of the disease.

CLASSIFICATION

I. Proposed by Ueno et al. and Later Modified by Lupi Herrera

- Type I: (Shimizo-Sano) Involvement of the aortic arch and its branches.
- Type II: (Kimoto) Involves thoracoabdominal aorta, but spares arch.
- Type III: (Inada) Features of I and II.
- Type IV: Pulmonary artery involvement (Right upper lobar artery and its segmental branches)
- Type V: Involvement of more peripheral vessels with sparing of the aorta (coronary artery involvement is considered type V by some).

II. Takayasu Conference 1994

- Type I: Branches of the arch
- Type II a: Ascending aorta, arch and branches
  b- ascending aorta, arch and branches +descending thoracic aorta
- Type III: Descending thoracic aorta + abdominal aorta and/or renals
- Type IV: Abdominal aorta and/or renals
- Type V: Diffuse-ascending aorta, arch and branches descending thoracic aorta, abdominal aorta and/or renals.

C and P represent coronary and pulmonary, their involvement indicated by +/- as the case may be.

CLINICAL FEATURES

Male-female ratio is about 1:8. In India, the female preponderance is less marked (M:F 1:1.6). The onset is in teenage years in 75% of cases. The mean age at diagnosis is 29 years. The presenting features in the decreasing order of frequency include:

- Hypertension: BP ≥140/90 mm Hg brachial or ≥ 160/90 mm Hg popliteal.
  Due to—
  - Renal artery stenosis
  - Aortic obstruction
  - Decreased aortic distensibility
  - Decreased baroreceptor reactivity.
- Constitutional Symptoms
  Fever, anorexia, malaise, weight loss, night sweats, arthralgia, pleuritic pain, fatigue, pain and tenderness over affected arteries.
- Features of Vascular Insufficiency
- Congestine heart failure (CHF)
  Due to:
  - Hypertension
  - Aortic regurgitation (occurs in 25%)
  - Coronary artery involvement usually of the ostia and the proximal part
  - Myocarditis
  - Cardiomyopathy-like picture in about 5%.
- Retinopathy: Usually associated with carotid artery involvement.
- Systemic Manifestations
  - *Renal*: Vascular—renal artery stenosis
    - Glomerular-mesangioproliferative—commonest, membranoproliferative crescentric
    - Amyloidosis
- *Dermatologic:* Erythema nodosum (commonest), ulcerated, subacute nodular lesions, erythema induratum,

papulonecrotic eruptions, papular erythematous lesions of the hands, facial lupus rash, erythema multiforme.
- *Cardiac:* Hypertension, aortic regurgitation, coronary artery involvement, myocarditis, pericarditis, pulmonary hypertension, dilated cardiomyopathy, congestive heart failure
- *Pulmonary:* Vascular - pulmonary hypertension, non-vascular - acute interstitial pneumonia, interstitial pulmonary fibrosis
- *Gastrointestinal:* Nausea, vomiting and weight loss (15%), inflammatory bowel disease.
- *Neurological:* Headache, paraesthesia, visual disturbances, Syncope, hemiplegia, seizures, hypertensive encephalopathy, paraplegia, Takayasu's retinopathy.

CRITERIA FOR DIAGNOSIS

The three sets of criteria are as follows:[1]
1. Ishikawa's criteria (Table 1)
2. American College of Rheumatology (ACR) criteria (Table 2)[8]
3. Sharma's criteria (Table 3).[2,3,7,9]

Table 1
Ishikawa's criteria

Criteria	Definition
Obligatory Criterion Age <40 year	Age <40 year at diagnosis or at onset of characteristic signs and symptoms of 1 month duration in patient history
Two major criteria 1. Left mid-subclavian artery	1 cm proximal to the left vertebral artery orifice to that 3 cm distal to the orifice determined by angiography
2. Right mid-subclavian artery lesion	The most severe stenosis or occlusion present in the mid-portion from the right vertebral artery orifice to the point 3 cm distal to the orifice determined by angiography
Nine minor criteria 1. High ESR	Unexplained high ESR >20 mm/hour (Westergren)
2. Carotid artery tenderness	Unilateral or bilateral tenderness of common carotid arteries by physician palpation; neck muscle tenderness is unacceptable
3. Hypertension	Persistent blood pressure >140/90 mm Hg brachial or >160/90 mm Hg popliteal at age <40 year. Or presence of the history at age <40 year
4. Aortic regurgitation or Annuloaortic ectasia	By auscultation or Doppler echo or angiography By angiography or two dimensional echocardiography

Contd...

Contd...

Criteria	Definition
5. Pulmonary artery lesion	Lobar or segmental arterial occlusion or equivalent determined by angiography or perfusion scintigraphy or presence of stenosis, aneurysm, luminal irregularity or any combination in pulmonary trunk or in unilateral or bilateral pulmonary arteries determined by angiography
6. Left mid common carotid lesion	Presence of the most severe stenosis or occlusion in the mid portion of 5 cm in length from the point 2 cm distal to its orifice determined by angiography
7. Distal brachiocephalic trunk lesion	Presence of the most severe stenosis or occlusion in the distal third, lesion determined by angiography
8. Descending thoracic aorta lesion	Narrowing, dilatation or aneurysm, luminal irregularity or any lesion combination determined by angiography; tortuosity alone is unacceptable
9. Abdominal aorta lesion	Narrowing, dilatation or aneurysm, luminal irregularity or any combination and absence of lesion in aorto-iliac region consisting of 2 cm of terminal aorta and bilateral common iliac arteries determined by angiography; tortuosity alone is unacceptable

- The proposed criteria consist of **one obligatory criterion**, two major criteria and nine minor criteria. In addition to the obligatory criterion, the presence of two major criteria, or one major and two or more minor criteria or four more minor criteria suggests a high probability of the presence of Takayasu's disease.

Table 2
American College of Rheumatology criteria (1990)

Criteria	Definition
Age at disease onset in years	Development of symptoms or findings related to Takayasu arteritis at age <40 years
Claudication of extremities	Development and worsening of fatigue and discomfort in muscles of one or more extremity while in use, especially the upper extremities
Decreased brachial artery pulse	Decreased pulsation of one or both brachial arteries
BP difference > 10 mm Hg	Difference of > 10 mm Hg in systolic blood pressure between arms
Bruit over subclavian arteries or aorta	Bruit audible on auscultation over one or both subclavian arteries or abdominal aorta

Contd...

Contd...

Criteria	Definition
Arteriogram abnormality	Arteriographic narrowing or occlusion of the entire aorta, its primary branches, or large arteries in the proximal upper or lower extremities, not due to arteriosclerosis, fibromuscular dysplasia, or similar causes; changes usually focal or segmental.

For purposes of classification, a patient shall be said to have Takayasu arteritis if at least three of these six criteria are present. The presence of any three or more criteria yields a sensitivity of 90.5% and a specificity of 97.8% BP = blood pressure (systolic) difference between arms.

Presence of two major or one major and two minor criteria or four minor criteria suggests a high probability of Takayasu arteritis.

Table 3
Modified diagnostic citeria (Sharma et al. 1995)

Three major criteria: 1. Left mid-subclavian artery lesion	The most severe stenosis or occlusion present in the mid-portion from the point 1cm proximal to the vertebral artery orifice up to that 3cm distal to the orifice determined by angiography
2. Right mid-subclavian artery lesion	The most severe stenosis or occlusion present in the mid-portion from the right vertebral artery orifice to the point 3 cm distal to orifice determined by angiography
3. Characteristic signs and symptoms of at least one month duration	These include limb claudication, pulselessness or pulse differences in limbs, an unobtainable or significant blood presence difference (>10 mm Hg systolic blood presence difference in limb), fever, neck pain, transient amaurosis, blurred vision, syncope, dyspnea or palpitations
Ten minor criteria: 1. High ESR	Unexplained persistent high ESR >20mm/hour (Westergren) at diagnosis or presence of the evidence in patient's history
2. Carotid artery tenderness	Unilateral or bilateral tenderness of common carotid arteries on palpation. Neck muscle tenderness is unacceptable.
3. Hypertension	Persistent blood pressure >140/90 mm Hg brachial or >160/90 mm Hg popliteal
4. Aortic regurgitation or Annuloaortic ectasia	By auscultation or Doppler echocardiography or angiography By angiography or two-dimensional echocardiography

Contd...

Contd...

5. Pulmonary artery lesion	Lobar or segmental arterial occlusion or equivalent determined by angiography or perfusion scintigraphy, or presence of stenosis, aneurysm, luminal irregularity or any combination in pulmonary trunk or in unilateral or bilateral pulmonary arteries determined by angiography
6. Left mid common carotid lesion	Presence of the most severe stenosis or occlusion in the mid-portion of 5 cm in length from the point 2 cm distal to its orifice determined by angiography
7. Distal brachiocephalic trunk lesion	Presence of the most severe stenosis or occlusion in the distal third determined by angiography
8. Descending thoracic aorta lesion	Narrowing, dilatation or aneurysm, luminal irregularity or any combination determined by angiography; tortuosity alone is unacceptable
9. Abdominal aorta lesion	Narrowing, dilatation or aneurysm, luminal irregularity or aneurysm combination.
10. Coronary artery lesion	Documented on angiography below the age of 30 years in the absence of risk factors like hyperlipidemia or diabetes mellitus

In a companion of the three sets of diagnostic criteria for Takayasu's arteritis, it was found that among Indian patients, the sensitivity and specificity of each of the three were as follows:

	Sensitivity (%)	Specificity (%)
Ishikawa	60.4	95
ACR	77.4	95
Sharma	92.5	95

NATURAL HISTORY

There are four patterns of disease noted they are:
A: Insidious onset followed by a plateau
B: Sudden onset of severe symptoms followed by decrescendo course
C: Early and late periods of severe symptoms with no severe symptoms in between
D: Crescendo course after initial plateau.

Complications

The four major complications as described by Ishikawa include:
1. Retinopathy—more than grade 2 (Uyama - Asayama).
2. Severe hypertension—brachial $\geq$200/110 mm Hg; popliteal $\geq$230/110 mm Hg.

3. Aortic regurgitation—grade 3 or 4 (Seller's angiographic grading).
4. Aortic or arterial aneurysms.

UYAMA AND ASAYAMA CLASSIFICATION OF RETINOPATHY

Stage I   : Dilatation of small vessels
Stage II   : Microaneurysms
Stage III : Wreath-like arteriovenous anastomosis around optic papillae
Stage IV   : Complications—
- Anterior segment—cataract, rubeosis and decreased intraocular pressure
- Posterior segment—retinal ischemia, neovascularisation, proliferative retinopathy, vitreous haemorrhage

Based on the severity of the disease, risk stratification is as follows:

Group I: No complication   low risk
Group II: a - Mild or moderate single complication low risk
         b - Severe single complication   high risk
Group III: 2 or more complications   high risk

ASSESSMENT OF DISEASE ACTIVITY

- Systemic Vascular Disorders Research Committee of the Ministry of Health and Welfare of Japan Criteria
  - Fever
  - Pain of vascular origin
  - Elevated ESR or CRP.
- National Institute of Health criteria: New onset or worsening of at least 2 features
- Vascular ischemia or inflammation, either extremity claudication, decreased or absent extremity pulse or blood pressure, bruit, or vascular pain, e.g. carotodynia
- Angiographic abnormalities
- Systemic symptoms not attributable to other events, e.g. fever, polyarthralgia, polymyalgia elevated ESR.

Drawbacks of Existing Markers of Disease Activity

In about half of the NIH cohort, clinical parameters and nonspecific acute phase reactants were inadequate measures of disease activity. 56% of their patients had a persistently high ESR during periods of remission and among patients believed to be enjoying prolonged remission based on clinical parameters, 61% developed new lesions on angiographic evaluation over a median follow-up time of 17.5 months.

- Imaging
  - Helical CT angiopgraphy - enhancement of thickened aortic wall during the arterial phase and further enhancement during the late phase. However, further information is needed on the correlation between the degree of mural enhancement and severity of the disease.
  - MRI:
    - Aortic wall thickness >4 mm
    - Aortic mural enhancement equal to or greater than myocardial enhancement on T1-weighted images and aortic signal intensity equal to or greater than myocardial signal intensity on T2 images during contrast-enhanced MRI.

INVESTIGATIONS

- Those which help in diagnosis
- Those which help in assessing disease-activity.
  - **Angiography** is the gold standard in delineating the extent of involvement. MR angiography is promising but is hindered by the lack of ability to measure intraluminal pressure and gradients.
    Angiography
    - Irregular intimal surface
    - Stenosis/occlusion of aorta and/or its branches
    - Poststenotic dilatation
    - Aneurysm.
  - **The investigations which help in assessing disease activity**
    - Low grade leucocytosis
    - Mild anemia of chronic disease
    - Elevated IgM and IgG in >50% are also seen.
  - **Chest X-Ray:**
    - Aortic knob widening
      [Distance from left border of trachea to the left lateral margin of aorta: $\geq$3cm <40 years of age, $\geq$4cm >40 years of age]
    - Irregularity of left lateral margin of thoracic aorta
    - Focal decrease in pulmonary vascularity
    - Aortic calcification.

Differential Diagnosis of TA Versus Coarctation

	TA	Coarctation
Gender	Females	Male
Systemic symptoms	Present	None
Claudication	Marked	Slight

Disproportionate Muscle development	Absent	Present
Collaterals	Scanty	Marked
Bruit	Abdomen	Thoracic
Rib notching	Rare	Common

TREATMENT

- Medical
- Revascularization: Percutaneous and or Surgical

Medical Treatment

The cornerstone of medical treatment is **corticosteroids either alone or in combination with cytotoxic drugs**. Medical treatment can halt the progression of the disease in about half the patients so treated and can result in lesion regression. Given below is the **NIH protocol**.

- Prednisolone 1 mg/kg/day, reassess at 3 months, if inactive, taper to an alternate day regime over 4–8 weeks, continued on alternate day schedule for 6–12 months or longer, tapered and stopped.
- Add on drugs for active disease or relapse.
  - Oral Methotrexate 0.15–0.3 mg/kg/week. (Start with 15 mg/week, increase by 2.5 mg/week to a maximum of 25 mg/week.
  - OR oral azathioprine 1–3 mg/kg/day
  - OR cyclophosphamide 1–2 mg/kg/day.
- If corticosteroids cannot be tapered to an alternate day regime at 6 months or withdrawn at 1 year, cytotoxic drugs considered failed and patient maintained on low dose corticosteroids alone
- In patients who respond, continue cytotoxic drugs alone for a period of 1 year, taper (azathioprine and cyclophosphamide 25 mg/month and MTX 2.5 mg/month) and stop
- About 20% have inactive disease at presentation; of the patients with active disease, 60% achieve remission with steroids at least once. However, 50% of these patients relapse while 40% of patients (steroid-resistant and relapsed) treated with cytotoxic agents go into remission. Roughly 25% of patients fail to achieve remission; and 50% of patients who had gone into remission, have at least one relapse
- **Nowadays steroids plus methotrexate is started together. If MTX** cannot be tolerated then give Azathioprine. **Next step is to add MTX plus LEF**[9]
- In a study from France, they had used with TNF alpha antagonists or tocilizumab with a 3-year follow-up

and found that relapse free survival was higher with this biological treatment than DMARDS [(90% vs 58%) Circulation 2015; sept 9: Epub ahead of print].

Indications for Revascularization

- Hypertension in the setting of renal artery stenosis
- Extremity ischemia limiting routine activities
- Clinical features of cerebral ischemia and/or critical stenosis of at least three cerebral vessels
- Coronary artery stenosis leading to ischemia
- Aortic regurgitation of at least moderate severity.

Prognosis

Survival rate		Ishikawa	Sree chitra
At 5 years after diagnosis		89.7%	80.3%
Event-free survival at	– 5 years	86.8%	61.6%
	–10 years	–	61.6%
15 years survival no major complication			83%
major complication +		96%	67%

The long-term outcome is adversely affected by—
1. Presence of any of the four major complications
2. Progressive course
3. ESR $\geq$ 20 mm/1st hour.

Predictors of an Acute Event

- Severe form of the disease based on severity of complication
- Severe hypertension
- Cardiac involvement
- Acute event–CHF, CVA, blindness, massive hemoptysis, acute myocardial infarction.

Results of Intervention – DR George Joseph's series from CMC Vellore *(Ref: 16th International Vasculitis and ANCA workshop 2013 proceedings)*

- **Restenosis after intervention is common**: Many of them will require multisessions. The first restenotic rate is 53%. But multiple interventions on follow-up it comes down to 13%
- **Bidirectional approach is required:** For Subclavian and aortic lesions Dr George Joseph uses bidirectional approach for better results
- **Monthly tocilizumab** infusions is able to halt the restenotic process, at least in the short-term, in this group of patients after intervention according to him.

COARCTATION OF AORTA

- Coarctation is a Latin word meaning contracted/pressed
- Coarctation ridge represents the original wall of the distal left 6th arch
- It accounts for 5% of congenital HD
- Type of CoA
    - Distal to the left subclavian
    - Proximal to Left subclavian
    - Right subclavian arises distal to coarctation
- **Hemodynamic Theory**
  Intracardiac lesions that decrease the volume of left ventricular outflow promote the development of coarctation in the fetus because of reduced flow through the aortic isthmus (Normal isthmus flow in the fetus is only 10%). Thus, conditions, such as VSD or AS which reduce the aortic flow and can easily cause CoA
- Ductal tissue theory: Migration of ductal smooth muscle cells into periductal aorta is responsible for constriction at the site of CoA
- Collateral flow
    - Anterior: IMA to anterior inter coastals
    - Posterior: Thyrocervical branch gives rise to Transverse scapular which in turn anastomoses with Thoracodorsal and which is a branch of subscapular a branch of Axillary artery to posterior intercoastal
    - Rarely, vertebral–anterior spinal–para spinal
    - The most common collateral is arteria aberrans from subclaivan to beyond coarct segment.

PHYSICAL APPEARANCE

- Legs may be thinner compared to arms
- Look for Turner's.

Turner's syndrome

- Short stature
- Short neck with websbing
- Broad chest with widely placed nipples
- Small chin, large ears
- Short fourth metacarpals
- Hyperconvex nails.

Signs

- Radiofemoral delay: It is not late arrival, slow rate of rise to a delayed peak
- AR amplifies the femoral pulse and obscures the signs of CoA

- CoA amplifies the brachial pulse and obscures the signs of AS
- Apex: May be heaving
- Parasternal heave if PH is present
- Collateral artery pulsation in the inferior angle of the scapula
- Gallops if the patient is in heart failure
- Murmurs: Three systolic and two diastolic.
    - From collaterals: Late systolic murmur—crescendo decrescendo, delayed in onset and termination or delayed systolic murmur
    - From the coarct segment: A posterior murmur—fourth or fifth thoracic spine; in infancy if the diameter is less than 2.5 mm, you can get a continuous murmur.
    - Bicuspid AV: Systolic murmur in the aortic area.
- Associated anomalies
    - Bicuspid aortic valve 40%
    - Shone's complex
    - Mitral valve abnormalities
    - Two shunts: VSD—30%, PDA.

Chest X-Ray

Rib Notching

- Is seen between third and fifth ribs.
- Seldom seen before 6 years of age
- Anterior intercostal do not lie close to the anterior ribs and therefore do not notch them
- **Causes of rib notching**
  9 arterial, 1 venous and 2 AV
    - CoA—75% of cases
    - Aortic thrombosis
    - BT shunt
    - Pulseless disease
    - TOF
    - Absent Pulmonary artery
    - Valvar PS
    - Pseudo truncus
    - Emphysema
    - SVC obstruction
    - AV of chest wall
    - Pulmonary AVM.

Unilateral Rib Notching on Chest X-ray

- Left subclavian arises below the coarctation
- Right subclavian is below the coarctation.

Why rib notching occurs in posterior intercostal?
Flow is in the opposite direction and that **too excessive with the result they become tortuous**; the flow is through the posterior intercostal to DA. Note: excessive flow through these arteries can happen with high output as well.

Natural History

- Mean age at death is 34 years
- Heart failure, aortic rupture, infective endocarditis, and intracranial bleed were the causes of death.

Treatment

Indications for CoA Intervention (ESC guidelines 2010)
- Peak to peak (or maximum instantaneous) coarctation gradient ≥20 mm Hg
- 50% narrowing of the coarct segment when compared with the aorta at the level of diaphragm if the patient is hypertensive.

REFERENCES

1. Ishikawa K. Diagnostic approach and proposed criteria for the clinical diagnosis of Takayasu's arteriopathy. JACC. 1988; 12:964-72.
2. Kerr GS, Hallahan CW, et al. Takayasu arteritis. Ann of Int Med. 1994;120:919-29.
3. Sharma BK, Jain S, et al. Diagnostic criteria for Takayasu arteritis. IJC. 1996:54;S141-7.
4. Hata A, Noda M, et al. Angiographic findings of Takayasu arteritis - New classification. IJC. 1996;54:S155-63.
5. Subramanayam R, Joy J, Balakrishnan KG. Natural history of aortoarteritis. Circulation. 1989;80:429-37.
6. Hoffman GS. Treatment of resistant Takayasu's arteritis. Rheu Disease Clinics of North America. 1995;21:73-9.
7. Ishikawa K, Maetani S. Long-term outcome for 120 Japanese patients with Takayasu's disease. Circulation. 1994;90:1855-59.
8. Arend WP, Michel BA, Block DA, et al. The American College of Rheumatology 1990 criteria for the classification of Takayasu arteritis. Arthritis Rheum. 1990;33:1129-34.
9. Kesar, et al. Management of Takayasu arteritis. Rheumatology, 2013.

CHAPTER 22

Approach to Congenital Heart Disease

Jacob Jose

CHAPTER OUTLINE

- Genetic Aspects of Congenital Heart Disease
- Consanguinity
- Bedside Approach to Cyanotic Congenital Heart Disease

GENETIC ASPECTS OF CONGENITAL HEART DISEASE[1]

8 per 1000 live births. 10% of spontaneously aborted foetuses.

Consanguinity

India has a long tradition of consanguineous marriages, mainly uncle-niece marriage and first-cousin marriages. In a study done from Mysore of 144 children with CHD, they found the odds ratio of 2.76; 95% CI—1.64–4.63 for developing heart disease. The common ones they noticed in their study were ASD, PDA and TOF.[2] It is likely that autosomal recessive disorders are likely to result from consanguinity and Downs syndrome incidence is higher in this group.

Autosomal recessive single gene disorders (Page 623 of Moss 8th edition)

- Ellis van crevald
- Keutel syndrome
- McKusick Kaufaman
- Smith Lemli Opitz
- Simpson Golabi Behmel Syndrome.

FOLIC ACID AND CONGENITAL TREAT DISEASE (EUR HEART J 2009;DEC)

The data from this study is supportive of a role of folic acid during the periconceptional period to **reduce the risk of CHD by nearly 20%, with a 38% reduction in the rate of septal defects.** The optimal dose and method of intake of folic acid through supplemented food, multivitamins, or an isolated folic acid supplement remains unclear.

CHD can be considered under three headings:
1. Left to right shunts

2. Obstructive lesions
3. Cyanotic lesions.

Clinical Features of CHD

Left to Right Shunts

- Recurrent respiratory infections
- Increased sweating
- Failure to thrive
- Cardiomegaly
- Signs of heart failure
- Shunt and flow murmur
- CXR—plethora.

Obstructive Lesions

- Absence of cyanosis or history of recurrent infections
- Normal shape of precordium
- Forcible or heaving apex
- Delayed corresponding S2
- Ejection systolic murmur
- Absence of diastolic murmurs unless valvar stenosis is associated with leaking valve
- Normal-sized heart
- Ventricular hypertrophy.

Cyanotic Lesions

- Cyanosis, clubbing, polycythemia
- Cyanosis is a word derived from Greek meaning bluish condition. Clinically, these cardiac lesions can be grouped into six headings as shown in Table 1.

Medical complications of chronic cyanosis (ESC textbook 2nd edition, page 320)

- Hematological: RBC mass increased—Blood viscosity increased
- Hemostasis: Platelet count and function decreased
- Metabolic: Uric acid increased
- Renal: GFR reduced
- Orthopaedic: Scoliosis
- Skin: Acne, clubbing
- Infection: Cerebral abscess.

Table 1

Cyanotic lesions can be put under six headings

1.	PS with right left shunt at atrial level	*Critical PS /Ebsteins*
2.	PS + VSD - TOF physiology	*TOF/DORV/TGA/SV*
3.	Transposition physiology	*TGA*
4.	Eisenmenger	*Cyanosis and Pulmonary hypertension*

Contd...

Contd...

5.	Cyanosis without PS or PAH	*Cardiomegaly–TAPVC/single atrium* *No cardiomegaly–Pulmonary AVM SVC to LA*
6.	PH due to pulmonary venous obstruction	*TAPVC with obstruction*

Pulmanic stanosis with right to left shunt at atrial level
- Dominant a wave in JVP
- Cardiomegaly
- Parasternal impulse
- S_2 widely split
- S_3, S_4
- Pulmonary ejection murmur
- TR murmur.

Pulmanic stanosis with VSD–Fallot's Physiology
- JVP is usually normal
- Normal cardiac size
- Mild parasternal impulse
- Systolic thrill uncommon
- S_2 single
- Ejection systolic murmur
- Diastolic period clear, no S_3 or S_4.

Cyanosis with Increased Flow: Transposition Physiology
- Symptomatic in the neonatal period
- Cyanosis – mild to severe
- Failure thrive
- Congestive cardiac failure
- Cardiomegaly
- S_2 single, S_3, insignificant systolic murmur
- Cardiomegaly with increased pulmonary flow on CXR.

Cyanotic Heart Disease with continuous murmur
- PA VSD
- TOF with collateral
- TAPVC
- Pulmonary AVN
- PPS with right to left shunt
- Surgically created shunts.

Table 2
Time of onset of heart failure in congenital lesions[3]

Age	Lesion
Birth to 72 hours	Pulmonary, mitral and aortic atresias or critical stenosis
4 days to 1 week	Hypoplastic left or right syndromes
1 week to 1 month	Transposition complexes, EFE, coarctation
1- 2 months	Transposition, ECD, VSD, PDA, TAPVC
2 – 6 months	Transposition, ECD, VSD, PDA, TAPVC, AS, CoA

CCF as a general rule occurs in the first 3 months of life. If there is no CCF in the first year of life, it is unlikely to occur till the child is over 10 years or more.

Cardiovascular Malformations in Asplenia and Polysplenia Syndromes

Structure	Asplenia syndrome	Polysplenia syndrome
Systemic veins	Bilateral SVC (65%); single SVC usually right (35%)	Bilateral SVC (33%); single SVC right or left (66%)
	Normal IVC in all, but may be left-sided (35%); azygos continuation rarely seen	*Absent hepatic segment of IVC with azygos continuation right or left (85%)
	Juxtaposition of IVC and aorta common	Juxtaposition of IVC and aorta occasionally
Pulmonary Veins	*TAPVR with extracardiac connection (75%) and often with PV obstruction	†Normal PV return (50%); right PVs to right-sided atrium and left PVs to left-sided atrium (50%)
Atrium and atrial septum	Bilateral right atria (with bilateral sinus node)	Bilateral, left atria
	Absent coronary sinus	Absent coronary sinus
	† Primum ASD (100%), secundum ASD (66%)	Single atrium, primum ASD (60%), or secundum ASD (25%)
AV valve	* Single AV valve (90%)	Normal AV valve (50%); single AV valve (15%)
Ventricles and cardiac apex	† Single ventricle (50%) usually morphologic RV or undetermined; two ventricles (50%)	* Two ventricles usually present; VSD (65%); DORV (20%)
	Left apex (60%); right apex (40%)	Left apex (60%); right apex (40%)
Great arteries	*Either D- or L-transposition (70%)	†Normal great arteries (85%); transposition (15%)

Contd...

Contd...

Structure	Asplenia syndrome	Polysplenia syndrome
	†Stenosis (40%) or atresia (40%) of pulmonary valve	Normal pulmonary valve (60%); PS or pulmonary atresia (40%)
ECG	Normal P axis or in the +90 to +180 degree quadrant	† Superior P axis (70%)

* Extremely important differentiating points.
† Important differentiating points
IVC – Inferior vena cava
SVC – Superior vena cava
TAPVR – Total anomalous pulmonary venous return

Role of Hyperoxia Test

This test is useful in differentiating from cardiac and pulmonary causes of cyanosis. Patient is given 100% oxygen for 10 minutes using a hood or endotracheal tube. Arterial blood gas to be obtained. In patients with cyanotic heart disease, paO2 rarely exceeds more than 150 mm Hg.

Teratogens

These are chemical or biological agents that can cause congenital anomalies. The Table 3 summarizes the same.

Table 3
Teratogen and cardiac anomaly

Teratogen	Abnormality
Fetal alcohol	VSD, ASD, TOF
Hydantoin	VSD, PS, TOF
Trimethadione	Combined defects
Valproate	Nonspecific
Retionoic acid	Cono truncal
Lithium	Ebsteins
Thalidomide	Cono truncal
Warfarin	PDA, peripheral pulmonary stenosis
Maternal diabetes	Transposition
Maternal Rubella	PDA, peripheral PS

Table 4
Common syndromes associated with CHD due to single gene defects[4]

Syndrome	Cardiac anomaly	Clinical features
Noonan	PS, HCM, AVSD, CoA	Short stature, Webbed neck, Shield chest, abnormal face
Castello	PS, HCM	Short stature, Developmental delay
LEOPARD	PS	Hypertelorism, deafness,
Alagille	PS, TOF, ASD, PPS	Bile duct paucity, typical face, ocular abnormalities
Marfans	Aortic root, MVP	Tall stature, etc.
Holt Oram	ASD, VSD, AVSD	Radial ray malformation- thumb, radial dysplasia
CHAR	PDA	Dysmorphic face, digit abnormalities
CHARGE	ASD, VSD	Coloboma, Chonal atresia, developmental delay

BEDSIDE APPROACH TO CYANOTIC CONGENITAL HEART DISEASE[5]

Table 5
Differential diagnosis of six groups

PS with Right to Left Atrial Level	• Prominent A wave JVP • Parasternal Heave • Cardiomegaly • Cyanosis Mild • TR may be present • ECG: RVH with Late transition	Critical PS
	• Quiet Precardium • Heart size increased • Multiple sounds • Scratchy systolic murmur • ECG typical	Ebstein's
PS with Right to Left Ventricular Level TOF physiology	• No cardiomegaly • Mild parasternal lift • Second sound single • Heart not enlarged • CXR: MPA absent decreased flow	TOF Physiology RAD RVH: TOF, DORV, TGA and SV RAD LVH : SV, Hypoplastic RV LAD, RVH: SV, ECD with PS LAD, LVH: TA, SV

Contd...

Contd...

Increased PBF TGA Physiology	Neonate or infant Failure to thrive Congestive heart failure Cardiomegaly CXR: Pulmonary plethora	D TGA, DORV, TA, Truncus, SV
PAH with No PVH Eisenmenger Physiology		Eisenmenger
PH with PVH		Hypoplastic left heart TAPVC with obstruction
No PS or PH	Cardiomegaly present	TAPVC single atrium
	Cardiomegaly absent	SVC to LA Pulmonary AVM

Table 6

Recurrence risk for normal parents and one affected offspring for non syndromic CHD[6]

Condition	Recurrence risk - %
ASD	3
VSD	4
TOF	2.5 to 3
PS	2.7
TGA	1
CTGA	5.8%
Tricuspid atresia	1
Ebsteins	1

When a second child does develop a heart disease, it is not the same type of CHD usually. The concordance rates are for VSD—55%, aortic stenosis 33% and coarctation 13%.

The risk of recurrence is greater if the mother has a heart disease by 3-fold. Higher risks have been noted for families with left heart obstructive lesions, such as coarctation, aortic stenosis or hypoplastic left heart syndrome.

Table 7:

Estimated risk of occurrence if parent had congenital heart disease

Condition	Recurrence risk - %
ASD	3
VSD	4
TOF	2.5 to 3

Contd...

Contd...

Condition	Recurrence risk - %
PS	2.7
TGA	1
CTGA	5.8%
Tricuspid atresia	1
Ebsteins	1

Table 8
Estimated frequency of CHD in 22q 11 deletion

CHD	Frequency %
Interrupted arch	50–80
Truncus	34–40
Isolated arch anomalies	24
TOF	15
DORV	<5
TGA	1

KEY POINTS ON GENETIC ASPECTS

- Chromosomal abnormalities are seen in 5-15% of CHD
- Cardiovascular anomalies are seen in 85% of 22q 11 deletion
- The most common abnormality seen with 7q11.23 deletion is supravalvar AS and Williams Beuren Syndrome
- In Noonan's—90% will have Valvar PS
- In Holt Oram—85% will have Cardiac abnormality (ASD and muscular VSD's)
- 70% of all CHD are isolated—nonsyndromic
- Recurrence risk in nonsyndromic CHD is 1-5%.

REFERENCES

1. Srivastava D. Developmental and genetic aspects of congenital heart disease. Current opinion in Cardiology. 1999;14:263.
2. Smitha and Ramachandra. Parental consanguinity increases congenital heart diseases in South India. Annals of Human Biology. 2006;33(5/6):519-28.
3. Tandon, Assessment of Severity; Chapter 10. Bedside approach in the diagnosis of Congenital Heart Disease. B.I. Churchill Livingstone Pvt. Ltd., New Delhi, 1998.
4. Genetics of congenital heart disease. Current Cardiology review. 2010;91-7.
5. Tandon. Bedside approach in the diagnosis of congenital heart disease, Publishers: BI Churchill Livingstone PVt Ltd. 1998.
6. Nora JJ, et al. Familial recurrence of congenital heart disease. Eur Pediatrics. 2007;166:111-6.

CHAPTER 23

Eisenmenger Syndrome

Jacob Jose, Parveen Kumar, Devi A

CHAPTER OUTLINE

- Definition
- Symptoms
- Signs
- ECG
- Differences Between the Groups
- Treatment

DEFINITION[1]

Pulmonary hypertension at systemic level due to high pulmonary vascular resistance over 10 units or 800 with reversed or bi-directional shunt.

ES Starts at Infancy in[2]

- PDA 80%
- VSD 83%
- ASD 8%.

Age at Presentation of ES

- 19 for PDA
- 22 for VSD
- 35 for ASD.

Size of the Defect and ES

- PDA   0.7 cm
- VSD   1.5 cm
- ASD   3.0 cm.

Ventricle Overload in ES

- Left ventricle in ASD
- Both the ventricles in VSD
- Right ventricle in PDA.

Prevalence of PH with CHD

- In a retrospective longitudinal cohort study of adult CHD from Canada, **5.8% had PH**. These persons had 2-fold higher risk for all-cause mortality[3]

- The major predictors of future PAH include the **location, size and complexity** of the native lesion. The risk of developing Eisenmenger's syndrome is **10–17% in patients with an ASD** (pretricuspid shunt), **50% with a VSD** (post-tricuspid shunt**), 90% of those with unrepaired AVSD** and almost all patients with truncus arteriosus.

Clinical Classification of Congenital Heart Disease (JACC Dec 2013)

Pulmonary hypertension associated with congenital heart disease

- **Eisenmenger Syndrome**
- **Left-to-right shunts**
  - Correctable
  - Noncorrectable
  - Include moderate to large defects; PVR is mildly to moderately increased systemic-to-pulmonary shunting is still prevalent, whereas cyanosis is not a feature
- **Pulmonary arterial hypertension (PAH) with coincidental congenital heart disease** Marked elevation in PVR in the presence of small cardiac defects, which themselves do not account for the development of elevated PVR; the clinical picture is very similar to idiopathic PAH. To close the defects is contraindicated.
- **Postoperative PAH**
  Congenital heart disease is repaired but PAH either persists immediately after surgery or recurs/develops months or years after surgery in the absence of significant postoperative hemodynamic lesions. The clinical phenotype is often aggressive.

SYMPTOMS

- **Dyspnea** on effort which increases with age; Patients with ASD and VSD have more symptoms than with PDA. Effort intolerance becomes increasingly common with advancing age, is more frequent in patients with ASD
- **Cyanosis** usually appears late and may be intermittent
- **Chest pain** is reported in 15–40 % of patients and is sometimes it is anginal in nature, occasional it can be pleuritic due to pulmonary infarctions.
- **Hemoptysis** 10–40%; in the later series it is only 6% and rarely in those under 20 years of age. It may be caused by **pulmonary infarction or rupture of a small thin dilation lesion** seen in the microcirculation.

SIGNS

- Cyanosis: ASD patients are cyanotic at an earlier age than VSD or PDA because of the ease of bidirectional shunting that can occur
- Clubbing
- Differential cyanosis in PDA
- JVP: Prominent a wave in 20–90% of patients. V wave is seen only in 5–20% of patients particularly in those who may have a LV to RA shunt or mitral regurgitation
- Heart is not enlarged but prominent PSL in most patients
- P2 is loud and palpable in two-thirds of patients.
- Ejection click—most patients
- EDM of PR one half to two thirds; 10% may have a thrill
- S_2 is single in 50% of VSD, 5–20% of PDA and 20% of ASD Wide split is rare in VSD, but common with ASD and PDA.

ECG

1. RVH 90% with ASD, 40–50% of VSD or PDA
2. RAE 20% common with ASD
3. Atrial flutter with ASD
4. Q waves[4]
   - Q waves in V6: 13% with ASD, and 33% with VSD 82% with PDA
   - Q waves in V5 and V6: 25% with VSD, 50% with PDA, rare with ASD.

DIFFERENCES BETWEEN THE GROUPS

Below is given the major differences between the groups

	ASD	VSD	Ductus
Angina	15%	14%	20%
Syncope	10%	14%	15%
Hemoptysis	25%	33%	12%
Congestive failure	10%	8%	12%
Squatting	5%	15%	3%
Sex	1:3	1:1	1:2
Effort tolerance	Grade 3	2–3	2
Cyanosis	75%	90%	33%
Differential cyanosis	–	–	50%
Dominant a	33%	Rare	Unusual
RV lift	Considerable	Slight to moderate	Slight to moderate
S2	Split	Single	Close split

Differences between the groups in chest X-ray and ECG

	ASD	VSD	PDA
Chest X-ray	Cardiomegaly Ascending aorta not prominent	Normal cardiac size Ascending aorta not prominent	Moderate cardiomegaly Ascending aorta may be prominent
ECG RAE RVH Q waves in V6 Q waves in V5, V6	Common 90% 13% Rare	Not common 50% 33% 25%	Not common 50% 82% 50%

A simplified differentiation between various groups has been suggested by Tandon[5]

	ASD	VSD	PDA
1. Cyanosis	Uniform	Uniform	Differential
2. Cardiomegaly	Present	Absent	Absent
3. Parasternal impulse	Heaving	Mild	Mild
4. Second sound	Wide, fixed split	Single	Normally split
5. Tricuspid regurgitation	Common	Rare	Rare
6. Ascending aorta in Chest X-ray	Normal	Normal	Prominent

Morphometric Grading

- Grade A: Abnormal extension of muscle into the peripheral arteries and the wall thickness is increased but less than 1.5 times the normal
- Grade B: Wall thickness more than 1.5 but less than 2
- Grade C: Artery numbers are decreased.

Alveloar Arterial Ratio

- Neonate 20:1
- 2 years—12:1 (Normal)
- Adult 6:1
- VSD PAH—25:1

How to Decide on Operability in CHD with PAH?
Criteria: With any of the vasodilators mentioned below, the net shunt should be left to right with—
- Fall **of mean pressure by 10 mm** of Hg to an absolute value of 40 or less
- Fall of pressure by 25% used for balloon occlusion for reactivity—useful in PDA.

Drugs used for vasodilator test:
1. Oxygen 100% for 10 minutes
2. Nitric oxide 5–20 ppm for 10 minutes
3. Isoprin
4. Adenosine 50 ug/kg/minute, increased by 50 ug/kg/minute every 2 minute to a maximum dose of 500ug/kg/minute.

Simple Methods to Decide on Operability[6]

For most post-tricuspid shunts we don't need a cardiac cath data to decide on operability. Simple methods as suggested may be more than enough (Table 1).

Table 1
Methods to decide on operability

Parameter	For operability	Clues for inoperability
Oxygen saturation	Normal 95%	Reduced 90–95%
Chest X-ray	Cardiomegaly, increased vascularity	Normal cardiac size, Reduced flow, Rapid decline in PA size to periphery
ECG	LV force with q waves	RV dominance, Absent q waves
Physical Exam	Flow MDM	Visible cyanosis, absence of flow murmur, EDM of PR

Criteria for closing shunts in PH with congenital heart defects (JACC 2013; 62: D34 – 41)

PVRi	PVR	Correctable
Less than 4	Less than 2- 3	Yes
More than 8	More than 4.6	No
4-8	2.3 to 4.6	Individualize

TREATMENT

- **Supplemental oxygen is not routinely recommended**: Patients who have significant desaturation with activity because of the increased oxygen extraction will benefit. The second group who may benefit is patients with right heart failure
- **Digoxin**: The efficacy of digoxin in this sitting remains controversial; however there have been reports of increased cardiac output with the use of digitalis in patients with pulmonary hypertension and right heart failure
- **Diuretics:** This drug is indicated in patients with right heart failure and volume overloaded. It should be done

cautiously to avoid over diuresis in these patients who rely heavily on preload to maintain adequate cardiac output.
- **Endothelin Receptor Antagonists**: Bosentan is initiated in ES in functional class III (class I, level of evidence B). The **BREATHE-5** (Bosentan Randomized Trial of Endothelin Antagonist-5) trial and its long-term open-label extension study demonstrated the benefit of Bosentan in patients with ES in terms of significant improvements in exercise capacity, hemodynamics and functional class compared with placebo, independently of the location of the septal defect. Importantly, treatment with Bosentan has been shown not to reduce systemic arterial blood oxygen saturation over short- and long-term treatment, demonstrating that it had no negative effect on the overall shunt. Treatment with Bosentan has also been shown to have a positive long-term effect on quality of life a particularly important consideration for Eisenmenger's syndrome patients. **Ambrisentan** is an oral once daily selective blocker for type A receptor. Trials: ARIES 1 and 2 and E. In the E trial, 383 patients were given the drug for more than 2 years. Sustained improvement was noted in the 6 minute walking distance. Liver function abnormalities were noted only in 2% of patients.[7] Tadalafil has also been studied in ES in a small group of 16 ES patients in a 12 week study with same results as other PDE inhibitors [8]
- **PDE5 inhibitors Sildenafil:** In an open-label study from China, this drug was given for 84 patients for more than 12 months and it was found that it improves the 6-minute walk distance, SaO2, in addition to the decrease in the PA pressure. [9] In another large double-blind study of 278 patients (Not all patients were ES) showed similar results.[10] The side effects due to sildenafil is shown in Figure 1 (**NEJM Nov, 2009**).

Role of Sildenafil in Children—FDA adds caution (Circulation 2012; 125: 324)

In a study done in children below the age of 17 years, a direct dose-related effect on mortality was observed with the highest dose having the worst outcome. The hazard ratio for high-dose compared to low-dose was 3.5 (p = 0.015). **Deaths were first observed after about 1 year, and then occurred at fairly constant rates within each group**. In light of these risks, the use of sildenafil **at high doses** is not recommended in children. A new warning against the use of sildenafil in pediatric patients is being added to the drug label

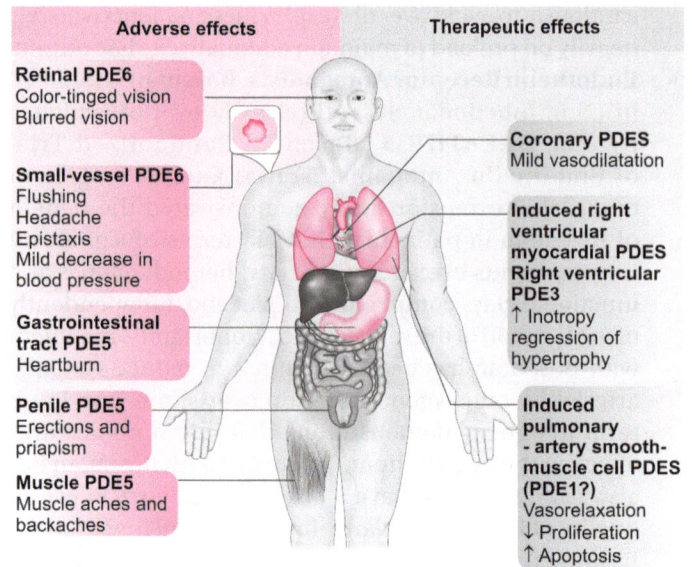

Figure 1: Sildenafil adverse and therapeutic effects (Adapted from NEJM)

- **Anticoagulation and antiplatelet drugs**: These drugs are **better avoided**, since they exacerbate the hemorrhagic diathesis
- **Calcium channel blockers are not used.**[11]
- **These should be avoided**:
  - Intravascular volume depletion
  - Heavy exertion
  - High altitude
  - Anesthesia and Surgery needs caution
  - Pregnancy.

  If a patient elects to continue pregnancy the following precautions need to be taken:
  - Admit the patient by 20 weeks till 2 weeks after delivery
  - Use epidural anaesthesia and cut short the second stage of labor
  - Heparin to be given during pregnancy and thereafter till discharge.
- **Lung transplantation** with repair of the cardiac defect or heart-lung transplant is an option for who have markers of a poor prognosis (Syncope, refractory right heart failure a high NYHA class or severe hypoxemia). **1-year survival after lung transplant is 55–70%**
- **Heart-lung transplant (HLT):** There are several limitations for this procedure. Patient with this syndrome have the highest perioperative mortality and the lowest one-month survival rates. Hence, this option is reserved for patients who are severely symptomatic despite treatment with optimal medical interventions. **HLT—1 year survival is 70%.**

Survival[12]

Patients with ES have reasonable intermediate survival with **many living to 3rd or 4th decades. Rate of Survival.**[13]
- 80% at 10 years
- 77 % at 15 years
- 42% at 25 years.

Survival of Treatment Naïve Patients with ES[14]

Based on 12 studies with a total of 1,131 patients, the mortality was estimated to be 30–40% for a 10 year period. This analysis challenges the traditional view of benign survival prospect of ES. The main reason for the quoted better survival is due to immortal time bias. To have correct idea on survival, we need to take a group of patients with CHD from birth to the time of development of ES and then to death which is not reported in most studies. In most of the reported studies, only those patients who have survived to an age with CHD and ES are enrolled in studies. This introduces bias into statistical analysis, leading to optimistic survival.

Suggested Treatment Algorithm for ES (Heart 2014;100:1322-1328)

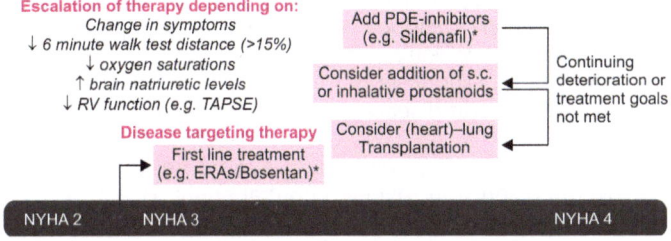

Table 7
Differences between ES and IPAH (EHJ 2014; 35: 691)

	Idiopathic PAH	Eisenmenger syndrome
RV dimensions	Dilation	Significant RVH
RV function	Rapid deterioration	Often preserved quite stable over time
Vasoreactivity	May have significant vasoreactivity	Minimal/no acute vasoreactivity
Prognosis without disease specific therapy	Poor	Often survive decades after diagnosis
Cyanosis prevalence	Late stages	The rule in Eisenmenger syndrome

Contd...

Contd...

	Idiopathic PAH	Eisenmenger syndrome
Cyanosis severity	Rarely severe at rest	Mild-severe at rest even in stable patients, severe on effort
Hematologic effect	Rare hematologic manifestations, Iron deficiency frequent	Secondary erythrocytosis common in Eisenmenger syndrom.
Systemic complications	Not common (late)	Common (renal dysfunction, gout, gallstones, etc.)
Associate genetic/chromosomal disorders	BMPR2 mutation in <25% of iPAH, low penetrance	Common (Down's syndrome)
Transplantation	Likely to benefit from transplantaion	Slow progression, not ideal candidates for transplantation

REFERENCES

1. Wood P. Eisenmenger's Syndrome. Diseases of the Heart and Circulation. 2nd edition. Asia publishing house; Bombay, 392-406.
2. Nihill MR. Clinical management of patients with pulmonary hypertension. Textbook of Moss and Adams, 5th Edition. William's and Wilkin's; 1695-1711.
3. Lowe, et al. Diagnosis of Pulmonary hypertension inn the congenital heart disease adult population. JACC. 2011;58: 538-46.
4. Wood P. The Eisenmenger's syndrome or pulmonary hypertension with reversed central shunt. British Medical Journal. 1958;5098-9.
5. Tandon. Congenital Heart Disease classification. Chapter 8 in Bedside approach in the diagnosis of Congenital Heart Disease, New Delhi; B.I. Churchill Livingstone Pvt. Ltd.; 1998.
6. Sangeetha Viswanathan, R Krishna Kumar. Assessment of operability for congenital cardiac shunts. Cath Cardiac Interventions. 2008; 71:665.
7. ARIES study group. JACC. 2009;54:1971-81.
8. Mukhopadhyay, Sharma M, Ramakrishnan S, et al. Phosphodiesterase 5 inhibitor in ES. Circulation. 2006;114:1807-10.
9. ZN Zhang, et al. Oral sildenafil for Eisenmenger syndrome. Heart. 2011;97:1876-81.
10. Galie N, et al. Silidinafil citrate therapy for pulmonary arterial hypertension. NEJM. 2005;353:2148.
11. Hawarth SG. Pulmonary Hypertension in the young. Heart. 2002;88:658-64.
12. Pediatric Cardiac Society of India. 2000.
13. Bricker MV, Hillis LD and Lange RA. Medical Progress: Congenital Heart Disease in adults. NEJM. 2000;340-6.
14. Diller GP, Kempny A, Inuzuka R, et al. Survival prospects of treatment naïve patients with Eisenmenger. Heart. 2014;100:1366-72.

Tetralogy of Fallot or Ventricular Septal Defect Plus Pulmonary Stenosis

CHAPTER 24

Jacob Jose

CHAPTER OUTLINE

- Anatomy
- Clinical Features
- Cyanosis
- Squatting
- Chest X-Ray
- ECG
- Oxymetry
- Angiogram
- Complications of TOF
- Differential Diagnosis
- Treatment of A Spell
- Catheter Interventions in TOF
- Surgery

ANATOMY

This malformation was reported by **Niles Stensen** in the year 1671. However, **Fallot** described the disease in detail in the year 1888 and published the same.

Tetralogy of Fallot (TOF) consists of the following **four** abnormalities:

1. Ventricular septal defect (VSD)
2. Pulmonary stenosis (PS)
3. Overriding of aorta
4. Left ventricular hypertrophy (LVH).

Spectrum of TOF Anatomy (% for Children's Hospital, Boston)

- TOF—66%
- TOF with Pulmonary atresia (PA with VSD)—33%
- TOF with Absent Pulmonary Valve (TOF with APV—3%)
- TOF with AV canal defect (TOF with AVC)—3%.

Embryology

All the above four components of TOF is the result of one morphogenetic abnormality—**malalignment of the infundibular septum.** Because the infundibular septum is deviated it encroaches on to the right ventricular outflow tract causing pulmonary stenosis, overriding of aorta and VSD.

Prevalence

As per BWIS Cohort, **5th most common** and the prevalence were 0.33 per 1000 live births. In other words, the overall prevalence is 1 in 3600 live births or **3 per 10,000 births.**

In a meta-analysis of 21 studies, it was noted to **have 557 per million births.**[1]

TOF occurs in 10% of all congenital heart defects. This is the most common cyanotic heart defect seen in children beyond infancy. The frequency in the siblings is 3% (If the father has TOF, the recurrence risk is 1.4% and for mother 2.6%).

Environmental Factors

- Maternal diabetes
- Retinoic acid
- Maternal phenylketonuria
- Trimethadione.

Association with Genetic Disorders

Increased frequency noted with consanguinity. Nearly 32 listed syndromes occur with TOF.

TOF is associated with a number of chromosomal disorders (nearly 20%) and they are listed below.
- **22q 11.2 deletion (**see below)
- **Down's syndrome**
- CHARGE
- Goldenhar syndrome.

The following genes have been (10%) have been described in literature
1. TBX5 causing **Holt Oram**
2. NOTCH1 causing **Alagille**

In 70% of cases, no gene abnormality is demonstrable.

Role of Karyotyping

In the clinical spectrum of **CATCH 22** syndrome (Cardiac defect, Abnormal facies, Thymic hypoplasia, Cleft palate, Hypocalcemia—neonatal), there is abnormality of 22q11, which can be detected by karyotyping.

Deletion of chromosome 22q11 can be identified in **15% of individuals**. Using Fluorescence in situ hybridization (**FISH test**) of peripheral lymphocytes, **only 2 spots are present**, whereas 4 spots should be present.

DiGeorge syndrome (DGS) now understood to be the chromosome 22q11.2 deletion syndrome was originally described as **3 syndromes**. Dr DiGeorge described the first of these 1965. Approximately 10 years later, in Japan, Kinouchi et al. described the **conotruncal anomalies face** (CTAF) syndrome, composed of congenital conotruncal cardiac anomalies, characteristic facies, learning dysfunction, and developmental delay. Shprintzen and colleagues in 1978 described their experiences in a craniofacial clinic with a syndrome of the same with special emphasis on velopharyngeal dysfunction with or without cleft palate, and learning dysfunction, which they termed the velocardiofacial syndrome (VCFS).

These individuals are more prone for mental retardation and schizophrenia in later life. There is a gradual decrease in IQ of these children.

Facial Features[2]

Eyes: Lateral displacement of the inner canthi. The palpebral fissures were short and sometimes narrow.
Nose: Bulbous-tipped nose and hypoplastic alae nasi.
Mouth: Small Mouth: The lips were thin in a third of cases with micrognathia.
Ears: The ears were low set and posteriorly rotated with deficient upper helices along with an increase in anteroposterior diameter giving a relatively **circular ear**.

Cardiac anomalies seen with 22q11.2 deletion
- 50% of interrupted arch
- 35% of truncus arteriosus
- 24% of isolated arch anomaly
- 15% of TOF
- 10% of VSD.

Reasons to test for 22q11.2 deletion before surgery
- Prone to develop hypocalcemia
- May develop GVHD and so need to give irradiated blood products

Types of VSD

- Subaortic—80%
- Subpulmonic—3%
- doubly committed—3%
- AV septal defect—2%
- Multiple—3–15%.

Morphologic Categories of RVOT Obstruction

1. Infundibular   26%
2. Infundibular + valvar   26%
3. Inf + valv + annular   16%
4. Diffuse hypoplasia   27%
5. Valvar stenosis   5%
6. Pulmonary artery stenosis   40%
    - Multiple level obstruction is the rule
    - A combination of infundibular and valvar stenosis was observed in 74% of cases seen GLH experience
    - Pulmonary artery stenosis—40% of cases and the origin of LPA may have narrowing at the ductus insertion site.

Haffman's Variant

It is a TOF, where the restrictive VSD is partially closed with tricuspid tissue, thus the RV pressure is suprasystemic.

Papillary Muscles of RV

In normal RV, there are three papillary muscles. The third one is small and attached to septum. In TOF, this may be absent. This muscle is called muscle of Lanseri.

Coronary Anomalies

- Entire LAD arising from RCA crossing the RVOT—4%—most frequent
- Single coronary artery from the left sinus is the 2nd most frequent – 1%.

Major Associated Cardiac Defects

- Right aortic arch—25%
- PDA
- Multiple VSD
- Complete AV canal
- Aortic valve incompetence
- RPA or LPA arising from the ascending aorta.

Minor Associated Anomalies

- ASD: 9%
- LSVC: 8%
- LAD from RCA 4%
- IAA 0.2%
- Aberrant origin of right subclavian 0.3%.

CLINICAL FEATURES

Pink Tets/TET

These children have minimal RVOTO at birth and they **may present with heart failure symptoms at 4–6 weeks** due to increased PBF due to fall in PVR and they shunt left to right.

Cyanosis[3]

25% are cyanotic at birth and 75% are cyanotic by 1 year of age. The late appearance of cyanosis is related to—
- Progressive increase in oxygen demand of the growing child
- Increasing PS
- After birth there is a slow change from HbF to HbA, which is a better carrier of oxygen than the later one.

Squatting

- With squatting systemic vascular resistance (SVR) increases and diverts the RV blood into the PA so that pulmonary blood flow increases
- Systemic venous return is even more important. Squatting decreases the venous return from leg, which has the lowest oxygen saturation.

Squatting Equivalents

- Squatting
- Sitting with legs drawn downwards
- Legs crossed while standing
- Mother holding infant with legs flexed upon
- Lying down.

Spell/Hypoxic Spell

- Increase in the depth of respiration
- Increasing cyanosis
- Hypotonia
- Syncope
- Seizures
- **Postspell somnolence is characteristic.**

Presentation of Spell

- Episodic loss of consciousness
- Episodes of going floppy/pale
- Episodes of going deeply cyanosed, loss of consciousness and sleep
- Episodes of rapid breathing
- **High-pitched cry.**

   Age at which spells occur: 6 month to 2 years in the early morning

   Duration of spell: 15 to 60 minutes

Precipitating Factor for Spell[4]

- Anemia—Hemoglobin should be more than 14 grams; moreover anemia will mask the cyanosis.

Murmur during Spell

The murmur becomes faint during the spell. However, in conditions, such as DORV, the murmur may be present because of obligatory shunt.

Complications of Spell

- Nasal speech
- Hypoxic brain damage and mental retardation.

Mechanism of Spell

- Wood's theory: Infundibular spasm; Catecholamine release leads to increased contractility and Infundibular narrowing
- Guntheroth's: Paroxysmal hyperpnea increases the venous return and more right to left shunt
- Kothari's: Mechanoreceptors in RV gets activated
- Morgan's: Vulnerable respiratory center
- Young's: Atrial Tachycardia.

Recurrent Respiratory Tract Infections

This is not a feature of TOF. However, in TOF with absent pulmonary valve, they can have this symptom and bronchiolitis, this is due to abnormal vessels entangling the bronchi.

Clubbing

PDGF released by the megakaryocytes that impact on the capillaries are responsible. If pain is a problem, Salsalate can be given, which is a non-acetylated analog of aspirin that does not interfere with platelet function.

Jugular Venous Pulse

The JVP is normal. In the JVP, **A** wave may become prominent in the following situations:
- Restrictive VSD—tricuspid leaflet tissue may partially occlude the VSD
- Hypertension
- Aortic stenosis
- Right heart failure—in adult TOF.

Precordial Palpation

- A gentle RV impulse in felt in the 4th and 5th LICS
- LV impulse is absent and the apex is formed by RV
- Right sternoclavicular junction may show an impulse in patients with right aortic arch
- Thrill may be palpable in the following situations: (a) If the RVOT obstruction is mild, (b) If valvar and infundibular PS is present, (c) If restrictive VSD is present.

Auscultation

Ejection Systolic Murmur

- The murmur originates at the zone of stenosis, not across the ventricular septal defect
- The murmur is equally prominent in the second and third left interspaces, but is typically maximum in the third inter space because the stenosis subvalvar

3. The length and loudness of murmur varies inversely with the severity of TOF. The relationship between the severity and the murmur are shown in Table 1:

Table 1
Relationship between murmurs and increasing severity of RVOT obstruction

Murmurs	Increasing severity of RVOT obstruction
Mild PS	VSD is holosystolic. P2 is delayed but readily heard
Moderate PS	VSD murmur declines in later systole; P2 delayed, softer
Severe PS	VSD murmur is replaced by a long PS murmur
Severe PS Exceeds SVR	RV blood is diverted–murmur shortens and softens
Very severe	Ejection click, A2 prominent; murmur very short
Pulmonary atresia	There is no murmur or only ejection click and collateral murmurs may be heard

- As the severity of TOF increases the murmur becomes shorter and softer. **Shortens** because infundibulum becomes more narrow in late systole. **Softer** because Right to left shunt increases with increasing stenosis
- Thrill is present in 75% of cases[5]

Second Heart Sound

P2 is soft or absent. P2 is soft because of decreased pulmonary blood flow. It is delayed or absent because of the delayed in the closure of the pulmonary valve due to pulmonary stenosis and delayed relaxation of the infundibular.

FEATURES OF ADULT TOF[6]

- Congestive heart failure—15%
- Hypertension—6.7%
- Aortic regurgitation—6.7%
- ECG may show LVH—0.7%
- Absence of RVH—3.4%
- q in lateral leads—8.8%.

Chest X-Ray

- PBF normal to be reduced; the middle and center two-third show no vascular markings. The main pulmonary segment is concave
- Cardiac size shows **boot-shaped heart**. This configuration results from the combination of a concave PA segment and a horizontal ventricular septum concaved by RVH, in the presence of LV that is smaller then normal. The left border is straight on top, rounder underneath, with an elevated blunt shoulder
- Right aortic arch is seen in 25%.

ECG

- Dominant R in V1
- Transition zone is in V2
  Reasons for the precardial pattern of QRS complex:
  – R is dominant in V1 due to RVH
  – S is dominant in V2 due to trabecular hypoplasia, i.e. presence of VSD
  – RS pattern in V3–V4 due to septal hypertrophy
  – S is dominant in V5, V6 due to LV hypoplasia.
- **P waves are typically peaked**, but are seldom increased in amplitude. The duration of the P wave is normal or short, because an underfilled and therefore, relatively small left atrium writes the terminal portion of the P wave. P is normal in height only in two-thirds of cases.[6] In 20% of patients, the P wave height may be 3 mm or more and this is especially seen in older children
- **QRS axis** downward and right; the mean axis is between +90 and +150. When right superior quarter axis is found you must suspect AV Septal type of VSD. Left axis is reserved for TOF with AV septal defect. In TOF with AVSD, ostium primum ASD is unusual
- **Depolarization** is clockwise with **an rS complex in lead 1** and prominent R in lead 2, 3
- **QRS duration** is normal
- T waves in right precordial leads are normal or inverted with equal frequency. Deeply inverted right precordial T waves that characterize severe PS with intact septum are uncommon because the RV pressure does not exceed the systemic level.

Relationship between axis and chamber hypertrophy in the differential diagnosis:
1. RAD, RVH - TOF, DORV, TGA, SV
2. RAD, LVH - SV, Hypoplastic RV
3. LAD, RVH - SV, ECD with PS
4. LAD, LVH - TA, SV.

ECG Axis

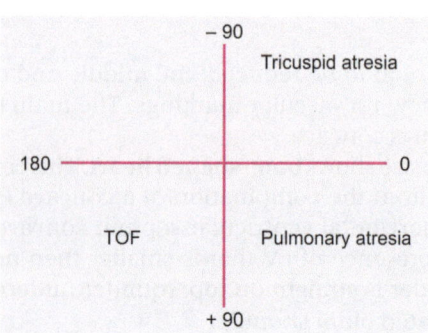

Oxymetry

- RA, RV and PA saturations are same
- PV saturation is near normal
- LA saturation is less than PV if Pentalogy of Fallot
- LV saturation same as LA
- Aortic saturation is more than RV and less than that of LV.

Angiogram

Cine is superior in detailing the PA anatomy, coronary anatomy and collateral flow. **MDCT is an alternative**.
- Look for additional VSD's—5%
- Look for coronary anomalies—5%
- Look for peripheral pulmonary Stenosis—28%.

COMPLICATIONS OF TOF[7]

- Brain abscess
- CVA
- Depressed IQ
- Scoliosis
- Gout
- Gallstones
- Infective Endocarditis.

Reason for cerebral abscess: Right to left shunts' bypasses the pulmonary filter.

Infective Endocarditis

IE involves the pulmonary valve commonly. Tricuspid valve involvement is less common. Aortic valve endocarditis is less common because LV empties directly into the aorta and thus there is not much turbulence at the site.

DIFFERENTIAL DIAGNOSIS
Within the VSD + PS Physiology

	TOF	DORV + PS	TGA +VSD PS	SV + PS
RV impulse	Confined to 4th and 5th LICS	Quiet, unsustained, confined to 4th and 5th LICS	Gentle RV impulse	
LV Impulse	Absent	Not palpable	Not palpable	LV impulse
Murmur	Murmur varies inversely with severity	Similar to TOF	Similar to TOF	Decrescendo systolic murmur, better heard in the lower left sternal border

Differences between VSD + PS versus PS with ASD

	VSD + PS	PS + ASD
1. Cyanosis	Almost all by 5–8 years	Late in childhood
2. Digital Erythema		May be present
3. Symptoms to cyanosis		Symptoms more than cyanosis
4. Spells	Common	Uncommon
5. JVP		
6. PSH		
7. Presystolic impulse		
8. Cardiomegaly		
9. Systolic thrill 2LICS		May be present
10. Ejection sound		Common
11. Murmur prominent		+
12. S4		+
13. S2	Single	Split
14. Chest X-ray: RAE	RAE is not a feature	RAE
15. ECG: RVH with strain		RVH with strain in V 1–V4

TREATMENT OF A SPELL

- Since most spells are provoked or worsened **by crying** the infant should be picked up, comforted, while being held in a **position of flexed knees and hips** that kinks the femoral artery and increases the peripheral resistance
- Knee-chest position in bed
- Oxygen
- IV fluid bolus administration—increase in intravascular volume and preload
- **Morphine** is the principle pharmacological agent used; the dose **is 0.1 mg/kg; can be given SC**
- Beta blocker: **Propranalol**, 0.01–0.25 mg/kg given intravenously; the average dose is **usually 0.05** mg/kg. ½ of the dose should be given rapidly under remainder slowly over the next few minutes (Esmolol 0.5 mg/kg as bolus)
- **Soda bicarbonate: 1 meq/kg IV**. The same dose can be repeated in 10-15 minutes. Soda bicarbonate reduces the respiratory center stimulating effect of acidosis. If the spells do not respond to the above four measures, the following medications can be tried.

- Ketamine: 1–3 mg/kg (average 2mg/kg) given IV over 60 seconds works very well. It increases the systemic vascular resistance and sedates the infant
- Phenylephrine (Neo-synephrine) 0.001 mg/kg given intravenously is quite effective
- Emergency shunt.

CATHETER INTERVENTIONS IN TOF

- Balloon dilatation of PS
- Balloon dilatation of blocked BT shunt
- Stenting of RVOT and infundibulum
- Transcatheter PVR in postoperative TOF
- Coil closure of MAPCA.

SURGERY

The diagnosis of TOF in general is an indication for repair.

- The appropriate age for ICR is **6 months,** if transannular patch and **9 months** if a transannular patch is not required. Nowadays, the age of surgery is around 3 months based on the experience of the center
- Shunt for before 6 months and **ICR between 6 months and 24 months** is not an ideal formula
- Two-stage repair is probably prudent for institutions not well-prepared for handling small kids.
- Primary repair should be the aim; when severe symptoms develop in the first 3 months an initial shunting followed by ICR within 12 months is a reasonable alternative.
- The surgical mortality is 4% if done with 1 year and 1.6% done around 5 years.
- ICR can be done by transventricular approach or transatrial approach or a combination of the same.

Primary Repair versus Palliation

- Kirklin et al. have concluded that primary repair without a transannular patch is as safe as a two stage procedure shunt—ICR, when the infant is more than 6 months and BSA is 0.35 sqm
- When a transannular patch is required, two stage procedure is safer if the infant is under 9 months old or has a BSA of less than 0.48 sqcm.

Annular Patch

- According to Kirklin, postopetative right to left ventricular pressure ratio ($P_{RV/LV}$) of <0.75 will be associated with a good functional result if VSD is adequately closed and the pulmonary valve ring is intact

2. If the $P_{RV/LV}$ ratio is > 0.75 intraoperative measurement of the pulmonary annulus by means of Hegar dilators has been used. A pulmonary valve annulus that is <50% of the diameter of the ascending aorta or less than a minimal acceptable diameter from a table of normal valves has been used an indication for transannular patch repair.
   - Z score more than -3: No need of repair transannular
   - Z score -3 to -7: Transannular repair can be done
   - Z score less than 7: Transannular repair not feasible, shunt surgery to be done.

Assessment of the Adequacy of PA Size

McGoon Ratio

Diameter of the right pulmonary artery and diameter of left pulmonary artery is divided by the size of descending thoracic aorta at the level of diaphragm. Normal McGoon ratio is 2–2.5. A ratio of more **than 1.2 is adequate** for ICR.

Nakata Index

This is the pulmonary artery **area index** assessed by cine angiogram. Patients with an index <60% of normal had severe problems with low cardiac output and congestive cardiac failure or died in the postoperative period. Normal is + 330 mm^2/m^2. Index should be more than 100.

Naito Index

This index is derived from left **ventricular end diastolic volume**. Patients with an index <30mL/m^2 are not adequate candidates for complete repair and should undergo palliative surgery.

Black Stone Formula

This is derived from diameter of right and left pulmonary artery and the pulmonary valve annulus measured from preoperative cine angiogram normalized to the patients descending thoracic aorta. This ratio should be >1.5:1.

Types of Shunts

- Classical **BT Shunt:** Done first in 1945; side opposite arch; subclavian artery dissected down and anastomosed to the side of the PA. Blalock was a vascular surgeon of John Hopkins who implemented the idea of a Pediatrician namely Taussig.
- **Modified BT**: It is side-to-side anastomosis; can also use Gortex conduit; can be done in small infants also. **Seroma** is long term complication of BT shunt.

In the literature, several complications of the m-BT shunts, such as thrombosis, aneurysm formation, hematoma and **perigraft seroma** were reported. The incidence has been reported as 6.8–9.5% following peripheral graft material
- **POTTS shunt (1946):** Descending aorta to LPA. Long-term follow up showed a significant incidence of pulmonary vascular disease. This has been given up but in patients with severe PAH, this was done to relieve the right heart failure
- **Waterston Shunt (1962):** Ascending aorta to RPA side to side; it may be the shunt of choice in small infants
- **Central shunt**: Gortex between ascending aorta to MPA. The flow is directed to both the PA
- **Classical Glenn:** SVC to RPA: End to end
- **Bidirectional Glenn:** End to side connection between the cranial end of SVC and RPA is created[8]
- **Kawashima Operation** is a further modification for those with bilateral SVCs. Each SVC is anastomosed to the ipsilateral pulmonary artery.

BT Shunt History

Many consider the description of this procedure, in the *Journal of the American Medical Association* (*JAMA*) in 1945, to have revolutionized the field of pediatric cardiology.

Helen Taussig, a pediatric cardiologist at Johns Hopkins at that time asked Blalock, surgeon whether he can create one ductus like surgery for TOF. **Blalock** had attempted to create an animal model for pulmonary hypertension through an anastomosis of the divided subclavian artery to the pulmonary artery. He was also attempting to treat coarctation of the aorta by turning the subclavian artery down and anastomosing it to the aorta below the area of the coarctation. A young African American surgical technician named Vivien Thomas was performing this work in an experimental laboratory. Thomas confirmed this in the laboratory, and Blalock finally performed the procedure on a 15-month-old child with severe cyanosis. Thomas alone had done all of the previous animal work (in >200 animals), and Blalock had practiced the procedure only once in the animal laboratory. During the surgery on the child, Blalock had Thomas stood behind him on a stool so that he could observe and instruct him accordingly.

Central Shunt

A central shunt is an anastomosis between the ascending aorta and the main pulmonary artery made of PTFE. The central shunt may be indicated in neonates **and children younger than 3 months**. It can be performed only in infants with a patent ductus arteriosus or some other source of pulmonary blood flow. A central shunt may be especially useful with bilateral small branch pulmonary arteries, a concomitant procedure requiring a median sternotomy, or both.

Watterson Shunt

The shunt is described as an end-to-side connection between a transected main pulmonary artery and the side of the ascending aorta.

Glenn Shunt

This is a connection between the SVC, and the right pulmonary artery end to side. The modification in current use is termed the **bidirectional Glenn** because it involves the connection of the SVC to the right pulmonary artery, which is still connected to the main pulmonary artery; hence, blood from the SVC can enter both the pulmonary arteries. One of its most significant **advantages** is that, unlike the other systemic to pulmonary shunts, it does not increase the volume load on the ventricle.

Repaired TOF

Long-term Complications Following Surgery

- Pulmonary Regurgitation—60–90%
- RVOT aneurysm
- Residual PS
- Residual VSD
- Aortic root dilatation with increasing age (Circulation 2013;127:172-179) 6.6% have increased size and the diameter may be more than 40 mm in adults in about 30%
- AR, which is usually mild
- Arrhythmias—sudden death—2%
- Heart failure.

Survival After Surgery[9]

- In one series, the rate of survival at **32** years after surgery was **86%** among patients with repaired TOF and 96% in an age matched control population. Ventricular arrhythmias can be detected in Holter in 40–50% with postoperative TOF. This is most likely to occur in patients who are older at the time of surgery and those with moderate or severe pulmonary regurgitation
- **Long-term survival is not the same** as of general population. At 30 years of age, a postoperative TOF patient has a **annual risk of death of 0.5%**.

Survival without Surgery

- 50 % at 3 years
- 25 % at 10 years
- 12 % at 20 years
- 6% at 30 years
- 3% at 40 years.

Causes of Death

- Spells
- CVA
- Infective endocarditis
- Cardiac failure
- Pulmonary hemorrhage.

Sudden Death[10]

The incidence of sudden death following surgery is around 1.5 per 1000 patients per year. **2%** of patients in the long run. (Lancet 2000; 356: 975)

- This event is likely related to ventricular arrhythmias or history of complete heart block
- More common when the patient was repaired at older age
- Moderate or severe LV dysfunction is more common
- **QRS duration of 180/msec $\geq$ and significant LV dysfunction are the greatest predictors for sudden death.**

Pulmonary Valve Replacement

Pulmonary valve replacement done for patients with RV end diastolic volume more than 200 mL/m² showed normalization of the RV volume within 6 months. If RV end-diastolic volume exceeds 150 mL/m² is used as a cutoff for patients following TOF, they should have good results.[11]

Indications for Pulmonary Valve Replacement (Geva. Journal of Cardiovascular Magnetic resonance, 2011;13:9)

In the presence of severe PR—regurgitation fraction ≥25% and

I. **Asymptomatic patient with two** or more of the following criteria
   - RV end-diastolic volume index: >150 mL/m2 or Z-score >4
   - RV end-systolic volume index >80 ml/m2
   - RV ejection fraction <47%
   - LV ejection fraction <55%
   - Large RVOT aneurysm
   - QRS duration >140 msecs
   - Sustained tachyarrhythmia related to right heart volume load

- Other hemodynamically significant abnormalities:
  - RVOT obstruction with RV systolic pressure ≥2/3 systemic
  - Severe branch pulmonary artery stenosis (<30% flow to affected lung)
  - ≥ Moderate tricuspid regurgitation
  - Left-to-right shunt from residual atrial or ventricular defects with shunt ratio of ≥1.5
  - Severe aortic regurgitation
  - Severe aortic dilatation (diameter ≥5 cm).

II. **Symptomatic Patients:** Symptoms and signs attributable to severe RV volume load documented by CMR or alternative imaging modality, fulfilling ≥1 of the quantitative criteria detailed above.

Examples of symptoms and signs include:
- Exercise intolerance not explained by extracardiac causes
- Signs and symptoms of heart failure
- Syncope attributable to arrhythmia.

III. **Special considerations**
- Due to higher risk of adverse clinical outcomes in patients who underwent
  TOF repair at age ≥3 years PVR may be considered if fulfill ≥1 of the quantitative criteria in section I
- Women with severe PR and RV dilatation and/or dysfunction may be at risk for pregnancy-related complications. Although no evidence is available to support benefit from pre-pregnancy PVR, the procedure may be considered if fulfilling ≥1 of the quantitative criteria in section I.

Summary Indications for PVR

Severe PR (Regurgitation fraction >25% of MRI and 2 of the following:
- RV EDV >160 mL/sq.cm
- RV ESV >70 mL/sq.cm
- RV EF <45%
- RVOT aneurysm.

Results of PVR

- In a study on 71 adult patients, it was noticed that **RV volumes decreased** by 28% and RVOT size reduced by 25% (Oosterhof et al. Circulation. 2007;116:545–551)
- In a study done on 98 patients, there was **no difference in VT or death**[12] (Circulation 2009)

Methods Used for PVR

- Stented bioprosthesis
- Hybrid procedure: Mini thoracotomy at 3 LICS: 29 mm stented 29 mm porcine valve through an incision of PA[13]
- Tissue valve replacement.

How to follow-up patients after TOF Surgery

- Infants and children up to 10 years of age yearly needs Echo
- Adults: MRI once in 3 years after the age of 10 years. Velocity encoded. MRI can accurately quantify the pulmonary regurgitation.[14] American society of Echo–ASE has laid down guidelines in the follow-up of patients after surgery for TOF which is given below.[15]

Modality	Age (y)				
	< 2 y	2–9	10–19	20–49	≥50
Echo-cardiography	12 mo	12 mo	24 mo	24 mo	24 mo
CMR	Not recommended routinely; ordered to address specific questions not answered by echocardiography		• 36 mo in stable patients • 12 mo if moderate (≥ 150 mL/m²) or progressive (increase of > 25 mL/m²) RV dilatation or dysfunction (RV EF ≤ 48% or ≥ 6% decrease in EF)		
CT	Not recommended routinely; ordered when CMR is indicated but cannot be performed (e.g., metallic artifacts or contraindications to CMR)				
Lung perfusion scan	If predicted RV systolic pressure 60% systemic or smallest branch PA diameter Z score < –2.5; in patients ≥ 10y of age, consider CMR flow measurements				

Contd...

Contd...

X-ray angiography	Not recommended routinely#: ordered when noninvasive methods either cannot be performed or have failed to provide satisfactory diagnostic data		Coronary angiography when clinically indicated
Chest radiography	Not recommended routinely; may be ordered for evaluation of stent integrity		

REFERENCES

1. Hoffman. The incidence of congenital heart disease. JACC. 2002;39:1890-1900.
2. Case of the month. J Medical Genetics. 1993;30:852-6.
3. Fyler DC. Tetralogy of Fallot. Nadas' Pediatric cardiology. 1992;30:471-92.
4. Pediatric Cardiac Society of India, 2000.
5. Wood P, Pulmonary stenosis with Dextroposed Aortic root (Fallot's Tetralogy). Diseases of the Heart and Circulation; Second, revised and enlarged edition. Asia Publishing House, 425-40.
6. Abraham KA, et al. Am J of Med. 1979;66:811-6.
7. Fyler DC. Tetralogy of Fallot. Nadas' Pediatric cardiology. 1992;30:471-92.
8. Hussain ST, et al. The bidirectional shunt: Interact CardioVasc Thorac Surg. 2007;6:77-82.
9. Bricker MV, Hillis LD and Lange RA. Medical Progress: Congenital Heart Disease in adults. NEJM. 2000;342:335-6.
10. Freedom RM. Congenital Heart Disease. Blackwell Publishing; 2004;207.
11. Buechel EV, et al. Remodeling of the RV after early pulmonary valve replacement in children with repaired TOF. European Heart Journal. 2005;26:2721-7.
12. Harrid DM, et al. Pulmonary valve replacement in tetralogy of Fallot: Impact on survival and ventricular tachycardia. Circulation. 2009;119:445-51.
13. Sven Dittrich. Hybrid pulmonary valve implantation. Annals of Thoracic Surgery. 2008;85:632-4.
14. Chowdhury U, et al. Annals of Thorac Surgery. 2006;81: 1436-42.
15. Multimodality imaging guidelines for patients with repaired TOF. JASE. 2014.

CHAPTER 25

Pulmonary Atresia with VSD

Jacob Jose

CHAPTER OUTLINE

- Incidence
- Morphology
- Environmental and Genetic Factors
- Embryology
- Pathology
- Classification
- Clinical
- Chest X-Ray
- MDCT
- Differential Diagnosis
- Natural History
- Management

INCIDENCE

- 2% of congenital heart disease
- 5 to 10% of TOF physiology.

MORPHOLOGY

In this condition, the following are the most important abnormalities seen.
- No blood passes from right ventricle to lungs. Hence all the pulmonary blood flow needs to be derived from alternate sources – see below.
- Pulmonary arterial anomalies are common
- Large collateral arteries are common.

ENVIRONMENTAL AND GENETIC FACTORS

- Maternal Diabetes (10-fold increase—BWIS cohort)
- Phenyl Keto Nuria (PKU)
- Retinoic acids
- Trimethadione
- 22q11.2 deletion in 10% of cases.

EMBRYOLOGY

- Lungs are developed from the foregut—in the neck and descends down to thorax; vascular supply is from pulmonary plexus supplied by intersegmental arteries. As the connection of the pulmonary plexus connects to 6th arch these segmental arteries disappear. **Failure of 6th**

arch development would logically result in persistence of the lung supply from the intersegmental arteries. **Hence, large collaterals that are seen in this condition are primitive inter segmental branches of dorsal aorta**
- **About day 27 of Embryo,** the arterial branches of the paired 6th aortic arches form an anastomosis with pulmonary vascular plexus. As a result the lungs have dual blood supply. With the branches from 6th arch enlarge and those from descending aorta become smaller. By day 50, the segmental arteries have involuted, so that the PBF is from the right ventricle.

PATHOLOGY

- **Right ventricular outflow:** In 70% individuals, there is **infundibular atresia.** The infundibulum is totally absent and the conal septum if present is fused with anterior RV free wall. In the remaining cases, there could be atresia of **RV-Pulmonary trunk junction.** The infundibulum is present but narrow. The obstruction is made up of thick membrane above the infundibulum
- **Pulmonary trunk:** Usually, the pulmonary trunk is present in 95% of patients, but hypoplastic. An unusual variation is that the pulmonary trunk may arise from proximal coronary artery system. Among patients with confluent RPA and LPA 10% have stenosis at its origin. An important feature is that these pulmonary arteries do not distribute to all 20 pulmonary vascular segments
- **Alternate sources of pulmonary blood flow:**
    - **Major aortopulmonary collateral arteries (MAPCA):** These are present in two-thirds of patients. These occur rarely in patients with TOF. MAPCA are large, 1-6 in number, they arise from the upper or mid descending thoracic aorta. They terminate with inter lobar or intralobar arteries. Extensive areas of intimal proliferation are present at the branching points or at the site of anastomosis so that 60% have stenosis
    - **Paramediastinal collaterals:** Usually arises from the subclavian on the opposite that of the arch
    - **Bronchial:** One on right and usually two on left. They arise from the thoracic aorta at the T3 to T8 levels with 70% from the T5 level. Right comes from the 3rd right posterior intercostal artery and it also called as Intercostobronchial trunk (ICBT). The left arises from the anterior thoracic aorta near the T5 vertebra level. The left superior one is usually lateral to the carina and posterior to left main bronchus. The left inferior bronchial artery is posterior to the left main bronchus.
    - Intercostal arteries

- **Coronaries:** Amin and coworkers found these type of collaterals in **10%** of patients with majority involving left coronary artery[1]
- **Ductus:** Is usually unilateral and is seen with confluent PA. Postnatal ductal narrowing will take place and so distal narrowing is present in 30–50% of cases.

Collateral Anatomy in PA VSD[2]

Three types of anastomosis:
Type 1 Bronchial → Intrapulmonary anastomosis
Type 2 Direct aortic → Hilar
Type 3 Indirect aortic → Extrapulmonary

Collateral Artery Supply Differences

	Bronchial	Direct aortic	Indirect aortic
Origin	Aorta	Descending Aorta	Descending Aorta/ Subclavian/ Coronary
Anastomosis	Intrapulmonary	Hilar	Extra-pulmonary
Course	Follow Bronchi	Distribution to segmental arteries	Variable
Embryology	When atresia develops later in gestation. These develop at 9th week of gestation after the paired intersegmental arteries are resorbed	Originate from the intersegmental branches of Dorsal aorta, which are normally present during 3rd and 4th week of gestation. Atresia at this time results in persistence of these arteries	Later in life

Differences between Ductus and MAPCA

Ductus	MAPCA
Widely patent at birth. Likely to have good-sized MPA	Small-sized MPA
Precarious source	Stable source
Postductal narrowing	Progressive stenosis
Normal distribution of PA within lung	Hyper-perfusion in some areas and Hypo-perfusion in other areas

CLASSIFICATION

Congenital Heart Surgery and Database Project Based on PA Anatomy

- Type A: Native PA present. No MAPCA
- Type B: Both native and MAPCA present
- Type C: Only MAPCA present.

Somerville Classification

- Type 1: Complete PA development
- Type 2: PA trunk atretic; with RPA and LPA present
- Type3: PA trunk and one PA atretic
- Type 4: Absence of PA trunk and both PA.

CLINICAL

- Infants with MAPCAs may have only mild cyanosis at birth. In the neonate, the continuous murmur may not be present at birth, but with fall of PVR after birth, continuous murmurs tend to appear by 6th week. In 25%, they may have CHF due to increased PBF
- There is frequently a continuous murmur from MAPCA, or a PDA. These murmurs are maximal over the side of the collateral at its point of stenosis and so they are heard right or left of the sternum or **posteriorly** because they **arise from the descending aorta**
- RVOT murmur is not present
- Normal S1 and single loud S2.

Chest X-Ray

- Coeur en sabot
- Right aortic arch in 50% of cases
- Pulmonary artery markings are reticular in appearance.

MULTIDETECTOR COMPUTED TOMOGRAPHY

Multidetector computed tomography (MDCT) modality is emerging as a good method to visualize the PA anatomy[3]

DIFFERENTIAL DIAGNOSIS

1. Pulmonary AV fistula:
    - The murmurs are typically less than grade III
    - 75% of the pulmonary AVM are in the lower lobe and in the right middle lobe, the murmurs are heard on these sides
    - Murmurs overlying the lingula of the left lung can be mistaken for intracardiac murmur

- The murmurs are prominent in systole
- Delayed in onset with a late crescendo
- Murmur may increase with inspiration.
2. **Total anomalous pulmonary venous recturm (TAPVC) with vertical vein:** A continuous murmur can be heard when the TAPVC connects with the left vertical vein and left innominate vein. The murmur as a quality of soft venous arm and is maximum at the upper left sternal border. Less commonly a continuous murmur is heard along the right upper sternal border where it is believe to originate from flow through a right-sided anomalous pulmonary venous channel into a right superior vena cava.
3. **Pulmonary artery stenosis:** The murmurs are usually typically confined to systole but exceptionally are continuous. It has been postulated that systolic expansion of the high pressure pulmonary trunk proximal to the stenosis sets the stage for brisk diastolic flow across the distal segments. Secondly, if the stenosis is severe bronchial collaterals may produce the continuous murmur.

NATURAL HISTORY

The survival rate without surgical repair is as low as 50% at 1-year of age and 8% at 10 years. Adult survivors of PA-VSD are quite rare. Marelli et al. reported that the mean life expectancy without operation did not exceed 3 decades, 4 and the oldest reported survivors were 54 years old.

There are three major subsets in relation to survival 5 (Crawford: 7.10.2)
1. **Confluent:** Normally distributing Right and Left PA 50 % of this category, 90 % die by 1 year.
2. Confluent but distribution is **not to all** pulmonary segments 25% belong to this category; 90% die within 10 years.
3. **Nonconfluent:** 25% belong to this category; these patients only mildly cyanotic, asymptomatic in the early childhood, good health till 15 years. Most of them are dead by 30 years.

MANAGEMENT

Palliative Surgery

- **Valve perforation:** If the atresia is limited to the pulmonary valve (e.g. imperforate pulmonary valve, membranous pulmonary atresia), the valve can be perforated percutaneously using special devices designed for this specific purpose, such as a needle or a radiofrequency ablation catheter. Then, after the

perforation is done, the valve is dilated with a balloon catheter. Stents can be placed in stenosed aortopulmonary collateral arteries in patients with hypoplastic pulmonary arteries
- Direct aortopulmonary shunts (e.g. Waterston shunt, Pott shunt) were used in the past, but not done nowadays because it causes distortion of PA anatomy. **Currently, the modified Blalock-Taussig shunt is used most commonly done**
- **Creation of a central aortopulmonary shunt:** For patients with confluent PA, a **Melbourne** shunt is created via an end to side, between PA and ascending aorta. For small central PA, 2 mm button is removed from the side of aorta, and connected. If the central PA is of intermediate type then PTFE tube is inserted between aorta and MPA
- **Valveless conduits or homografts** may be used to connect the right ventricle (RV) to the pulmonary artery. This may promote the growth of pulmonary arteries.
- **Banding:** In infants with CHF caused by excessive aortopulmonary collateral arteries, flow can be reduced by performing surgical interruption or by judicious banding or percutaneous coil occlusion of selected systemic arterial collaterals.

Intracardiac Repair

Criteria for complete surgical repair:
- If central pulmonary arteries are present, their central area must be more than 50% of normal for the patient's age and body surface area.
- The pulmonary arteries must supply at least 10 segments, the equivalent of one lung.
- If a single pulmonary artery is present, it must be normal in size and reach all segments of that lung.

Various approaches have been devised to achieve a complete surgical repair, including the following:
- **Single stage unifocalization and ICR:** If a patient meets all the criteria for complete repair done 4–8 months of age
- Single-stage unifocalization and postponement of ventricular septal defect closure to a second operation is an option
- Sequential unilateral unifocalization followed by intracardiac repair is preferred in some patients.

Treatment Based on Pulmonary Circulation[6]

PA-VSD Type A

Native PA present along with ductus—no MAPCA are Surgical options primary intracardiac repair is possible. Alternatively, an initial systemic-to-pulmonary shunt may be performed with intracardiac repair delayed to a later date. Pulmonary unifocalization is not required. However, creation of a pulmonary confluence between the RPA and LPA may be necessary if they are discontinuous.

PA-VSD Type B

Both native PA and MAPCA are present. Surgical options are—single-stage midline bilateral pulmonary unifocalization with concomitant or delayed intracardiac repair may be possible. Alternatively, a multistage surgical approach may consist of preliminary operations to develop the NPA, sequential unilateral pulmonary unifocalizations to centralize pulmonary blood flow, and finally followed by intracardiac repair, if the criteria for reparability are fulfilled.

PA-VSD Type C

There are no Native PA. Only MAPCAs are present: Surgical optionsare—single-stage midline bilateral pulmonary unifocalization with concomitant or delayed intracardiac repair may be possible. Alternatively, a multistage surgical approach may consist of preliminary operations to centralize pulmonary blood flow, such as sequential unilateral pulmonary unifocalizations, followed by intracardiac repair if the criteria for reparability are fulfilled.

Results of Surgery

- In a study of 85 patients with 1 stage unifocalization and ICR, they could do complete repair in two-thirds of patients even with absence of true PA. The actuarial survival was 80% at 3 years. The median age of repair was 7 months of age[7]
- In one report of late surgery in PAVSD, they could do complete repair in only 50% of patients. Many underwent only a palliative shunt and this improved their functional status[8]
- Large series from Cho et al. in 495 patients, in whom staged procedures were done, 68% could undergo complete repair eventually.

REFERENCES

1. Zahid Amin, et al. Coronary to pulmonary artery collaterals in patients with pulmonary atresia and ventricular septal defect. Ann Thora Sur. 2000;70:119-23.
2. Rabinovitch M. Growth and Development of the pulmonary vascular bed in patients with tetralogy of Fallot with or without pulmonary atresia. Circulation. 1981;64:1234.
3. Fukui D, et al. Longest survivor of PA VSD; Circulation. 2011; 124:2155-7.

4. Marelli AJ, Perloff JK, Child JS, Laks H. Pulmonary atresia with ventricular septal defect in adults. Circulation. 1994;89:243-51.
5. Murphy DJ and Mee RBB. Pulmonary atresia with ventricular septal defect. Crawford MH: Mosby;2001.7.10.2.
6. Tchervenkov CI, Roy N. Congenital Heart Surgery Nomenclature and Database project. Annals of Thoracic Surgery. 2000;69:s97-105.
7. Reddy VM, et al. Early and intermediate outcomes after repair of PA VSD. Circulation 2000;101:1826-32.
8. Belli E, et al. Surgical management of PA VSD in late adolescence and adulthood. European Journal of Cardio Thoracic surgery. 2007;31:236-41.

CHAPTER 26

Chest X-Ray

Jacob Jose, Parveen Kumar

CHAPTER OUTLINE

- Assessing Heart Size
- Left Atrium Enlargement
- Right Atrium
- Left Ventricle
- Right Ventricle
- Pulmonary Blood Flow

AP versus PA—Heart size

- The standard chest radiograph is taken with the patient standing up, and with the X-ray beam passing through the patient from **Posterior to Anterior** (PA)
- The chest X-ray image produced is viewed as if looking at the patient from the front, face-to-face. The heart is on the right side of the image as you look at it
- The heart, being an anterior structure within the chest, is **magnified by an AP view**. Magnification is exaggerated further by the shorter distance between the X-ray source and the patient, often required when acquiring an AP image. This leads to a more divergent beam to cover the same anatomical field
- As a rule of thumb, you should never consider the heart size to be enlarged if the projection used is AP. If however, the heart size is normal on an AP view, then you *can* say it is *not* enlarged.

Assessing Inspiration

- When interpreting a chest X-ray, it is important to recognize if there has been incomplete inspiration. If the image is acquired in the expiratory phase, the lungs are relatively airless and their density is increased. Also, the raised position of the diaphragm leads to exaggeration of heart size, and obscuration of the lung bases
- To assess the degree of inspiration, it is conventional to count anterior parts of ribs down to the diaphragm. The diaphragm should be intersected by **the 5th to 7th anterior ribs in the midclavicular line**. Less is a sign of incomplete inspiration.

Penetration

- Penetration is the degree to which X-rays have passed through the body. **A well-penetrated chest X-ray is one where the vertebrae are just visible behind the heart.**

ASSESSING HEART SIZE

- **Transverse Cardiac diameter**: 90% males less than 13.5 cm; 90% Females less than 12.5 cm between examinations, a variation of up to 1.5 cm is acceptable. More than 2 cm indicates increase in cardiac size
- *Cardiothoracic ratio:* Normal—50%; 55% for blacks & Asians; 60% neonates and elderly.
  This is difficult to assess in transverse and vertical hearts. The ratio is increased by faulty techniques like incomplete inspiration, supine, prone, anteroposterior view, and short-tube film distance. Selective chamber enlargement may be recognized on plain radiograph by the change in appearance it produces.
  - Affected chamber will expand, displace and deform the part of cardiac silhouette it forms
  - Affected chamber may appear in the cardiac silhouette in a view in which it is not normally seen
  - The enlarged chamber may cause recognizable displacement of contiguous structures.

LEFT ATRIUM ENLARGEMENT

- **Straightening** of the left heart border due to left atrial appendage filling up
- **Elevation of left main bronchus/Carinal Angle:** This will depend on the fact that whether LA enlargement did take place before the mediastinum is fixed as it happens with increasing age. The younger the age it is more likely to be seen. Carinal angle: **normal angle is up to 75 or** so; however, if it is more than 100, LA is definitely enlarged. Inspiration and timing of the cardiac cycle at which the CXR is taken can alter the carinal angle.
- **Shadow in shadow/double atrial shadow:** The left atrium is seen within the shadow of the right atrium
- **Right border formed by LA/LA forming right border:** This can happen with large LA and this happens laterally. Usually, seen with a combination of MS with MR. This is also called **as Atrial Escape**.
- **Giant Left atrium:** Left atrium touching the right chest wall.[1] Giant LA is defined as diameter of more than 65mm on Echo.[2] **For chest X-ray the right border should touch the right chest wall**

- **Oblique diameter >7 cm:** Measured from the **midinferior border** of left main bronchus to outer limit of LA on the right heart border. Highly reliable
- Displacement of descending thoracic aorta to left (Not reliable after 50 years of age because of unfolding of aorta) seen in 50–80%
- Displacement of barium-filled esophagus to right, rarely to left. Especially in children, this is better made out in RAO 30° and lateral views.

Causes of Double Density

- LA enlargement
- Aortic root enlargement
- Confluence of pulmonary veins.

Differentiating features of double density caused by a dilated LA compared to normal LA
1. The shadow is more inferior or horizontal
2. The radius of curvature is more
3. The distance from the middle of the right border of double density to the left main bronchus
    - Normal—less than 7 cm in 96% of individuals
    - More than 7 cm in females—abnormal
    - More than 7.5 cm in males—abnormal.

Causes of Elevation of Left Main Bronchus

- Cardiomegaly which is especially marked
- Pericardial effusion.

Causes of Enlargement of Left Atrial Appendage (LAA)

- Idiopathic dilatation of LAA
- Partial absence of pericardium
- Congenital diverticulum of LA.

RIGHT ATRIUM

- The right heart border extends for more than 5.5 cm from the midline or 3.5 cm from the right sternal border
- The vertical extent of the right atrium is 50% or more of the height of the right hemithorax.
- Right atrium spans over 2½ intercostal spaces in its vertical extend
- Increased curvature or radius of curvature of right heart border
- Step-like angle between RA and SVC.

LEFT VENTRICLE

In PA view, LV forms lower portion of left border and apex while in lateral view it forms the posterior aspect of cardiac silhouette below AV ring.

PA View

- Rounding of apex: This may be due to hypertrophy alone and may be recognized before significant enlargement
- Elongation of long axis of LV to the left and downward is earliest feature of dilatation. Apex may be shifted below diaphragm.

Lateral View

- Extension behind barium filled esophagus by more than 1.8 cm
- Displacement of posteroinferior border of heart to a point behind IVC at a point 2 cm above diaphragm (**Hoffman-Rigler sign**).

RIGHT VENTRICLE

Lateral View

- **Sternal contact sign—earliest and most sensitive**. This is always to be interpreted in relation to shape of chest, i.e. depressed sternum increases and bowed sternum decreases area of contact. Abnormalities of chest is common in congenital heart disease
- Increase in bulk of anterior portion of heart.

PA View

- Cardiac enlargement—broadening of the triangular-shaped RV. **LV is displaced upwards and outwards resulting in prominence of upper ventricular border**. With severe RV enlargement, it may form part of the left heart border. Left cardio phrenic angle is acute.
- Tilted up and posterior displacement of LV
- Corroborative evidence—prominent MPA, peripheral vessels may be increased/pruned/decreased.

PULMONARY BLOOD FLOW

Increased Pulmonary Vascularity

- PA branches are visualized far **beyond** the usual 2/3rd of the lung, field. The vessels in both the **upper and lower lobes** appear to be dilated to the same degree
- The number of end on vessels are **5 or more in both the lung fields or 3 or more in one lung** field
- End on vessels seen beyond 10th rib posteriorly
- End on vessels exceeding the diameter of the accompanying bronchus – AB ratio is more than 1
- The transverse diameter of the right descending pulmonary artery is more than the normal. 16 **mm or**

more is the usual cut off. Or more than the size of **trachea**. The normal value for males is 15 mm and in females 14 mm.

Pulmonary Artery Hypertension

- Peripheral pruning
- Marked dilatation of the MPA and the main pulmonary arteries.

Pulmonary Artery Stenosis

- The main pulmonary artery segment is dilated; this is due to poststenotic dilatation
- The left pulmonary artery is also dilated
- The pulmonary blood flow is usually normal or the vascular markings can be reduced in size.

Decreased Pulmonary Blood Flow

- The pulmonary vascular markings are markedly reduced.
- The pulmonary vessels in the middle 1/3rd and lateral 1/3rd are markedly attenuated.

Congestive Cardiac Failure

- ***Kerley B lines,*** distinct, parallel opacities in the lung bases, oriented perpendicular to the pleural surface
- **Kerley's C lines a**re reticular opacities at the lung base, representing Kerley's B lines *en face* (NEJM April 9, 2009)
- **Kerley's A lines (arrows**) are linear opacities extending from the periphery to the hila. *A lines* are the radiographic manifestation of more deeply situated lymphatic segments and appear as randomly distributed linear densities found in the **mid-lung fields**
- ***Cephalization of blood flow:*** In these cases, the caliber of an upper lobe pulmonary vessel is greater than that of another vessel measured from an equal distance from the pulmonary hilus in the lower lobe. This can happen in 3 situations:
  - Left heart failure
  - Left heart obstructions, such as mitral stenosis
  - Severe mitral regurgitation without LV failure.

  To call it cephalization, upper lobe vessels should be prominent with constriction of the lower lobe vessels. In left to right shunts there can be upper lobe vessels prominent without narrowing of the lower lobe vessels.
- In pulmonary edema, the alveolar air is replaced by edema. The confluent, patchy infiltrates of pulmonary edema usually involve the medial two-thirds of the lungs and expand outward from the mediastinum, giving the ***appearance of bat wings***

- The most frequent presentation of acute pulmonary edema is that of bilateral, fluffy pulmonary infiltrates
- The size of pulmonary vessel in the first intercostals space is more than 3 mm.

Grading of Pulmonary Venous Hypertension[3]

The grading of PVH is dependent on the distribution of vessels and the right hilar angle.

- Grade 1: The diameter of the vessels in the upper zone is either **equal** to or **greater** than those of the lower zone vessels. Right Hilar angle: the angle is concave normally and it is obliterated
- Grade 2: **Interstitial pulmonary** edema and pleural effusion. The most reliable signs are Kerley B lines. Kerley A lines are seen in acute or advanced degree or grade 2 PVH. In this, the right hilar angle is straightened
- Grade 3: **Alveolar edema**; the right hilar angle is convex

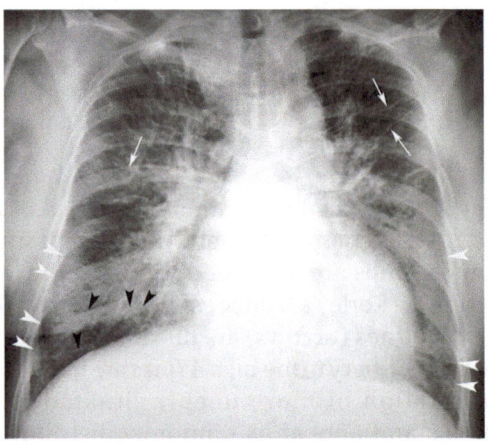

Figure 1: Kerley's A lines (arrows) are linear opacities extending from the periphery to the hila; they are caused by distention of anastomotic channels between peripheral and central lymphatics. Kerley's B lines (white arrowheads) are short horizontal lines situated perpendicularly to the pleural surface at the lung base; they represent edema of the interlobular septa. Kerley's C lines (black arrowheads) are reticular opacities at the lung base, representing Kerley's B lines en face
Source: NEJM Apr 09; Reproduced with permission

Grading of PVH and PCW

	Acute	*Chronic*
Grade 1	14–19	14–19
Grade 2	20–25	20–30
Grade 3	More than 25	More than 30

Pleural Effusion in Heart Failure

80% are bilateral and this closely related to interstitial edema—so more common with left heart failure than right heart failure. The effusion can be exudative as well if diuretics is being used. Serum effusion—albumin gradient <1.2 or serum—effusion total protein gradient <3.1 has better specificity to identify an exudative effusion in patients with heart failure.[4]

REFERENCES

1. Hurst: Circulation. 2002;105:e190.
2. European Journal Cardio Thoracic Surgery. 2008;182-90.
3. Grainger & Allison's. Diagnostic Radiology – A textbook of medical imaging. Churchill Livingstone. 2001;874-6.
4. Chest. 2002;122:1518.

CHAPTER 27

ECG Criterias

Parveen Kumar

CHAPTER OUTLINE

- Left Atrial Enlargement
- Right Atrial Enlargement
- Biatrial Enlargement
- Right Ventricular Hypertrophy
- Left Ventricular Hypertrophy: Voltage Criteria
- Stepwise Criteria Favoring Ventricular Tachycardia

LEFT ATRIAL ENLARGEMENT[1]

Criterion	Sensitivity	Specificity
1. P terminal force: Morris Index	69%	93%
2. Notched P wave in any standard lead with inter-peak duration >0.04 sec	15%	100%
3. P wave duration >0.12in in lead II	33%	88%
4. P wave duration/PR segment >1.6 in lead II: Macruz Index	31%	64%
6. Leftward shift of the P wave axis between −30 and +45 degrees		

Munuswamy et al. found that the most sensitive was increased duration of the terminal negative portion of the P wave and the most specific was wide notched P wave.[2]

RIGHT ATRIAL ENLARGEMENT

- qR morphology in V1 in the absence of infarction (specificity 100%)
- P wave more than 2.5 mm in lead II or more than 1.5 mm in V1
- Rightward shift of the mean P wave axis to above 75°
- V2/V1 QRS voltage ratio[3] 5 mm with QRS voltage in V1 <4 mm (specificity 90%)
- Early terminal negativity in V1< 0.03 second.

BIATRIAL ENLARGEMENT

- Large biphasic P in V1 with initial positive component 1.5 mm and P terminal force with negative component of 1mm and duration of 0.04 second.

- Tall P wave >1.5 mm in V1 to V3 and wide, notched P in left precordial leads V5-V6.

RIGHT VENTRICULAR HYPERTROPHY

		Amplitude
1.	Tall R V_1	>6 mm
2.	Increased R:S ratio V_1	>1.0
3.	Deep S V_5	>10 mm
4.	Deep S V_6	>3 mm
5.	R V_1+S $V_{5,6}$	>10.5 mm

Buttler and Legget Criteria for RVH

- P Wave amplitude >2.5 mm in any of the leads II, III, aVF, V1 or V2.
- R wave amplitude <2 mm in lead I.
- A + R – PL >7 mm where A (Anterior directed deflection) is derived from lead V1 or V2 R (Rightward deflection) is the S amplitude in lead I or V6 and PL (Posterolateral deflection) is S amplitude in V1.

LEFT VENTRICULAR HYPERTROPHY: VOLTAGE CRITERIA[3]

		Amplitude
1.	Limb lead voltage R aVL	>11 mm
2	Precordial lead voltage: S V_1+R V_5 S V_2+ R $V_{5,6}$	>35 mm >45 mm
3	Combinations of limb and precordial voltage Total 12-lead voltage	>175 mm
4	Criteria for use with left anterior fascicular block S V_1+R V_5+S V_5	>25
5	Criteria for use with RBBB: R $V_{5,6}$	>15 mm

Left Ventricular Hypertrophy—Romhilt-Estes Point Score System

Criterion	
Amplitude :Any of the following: Any limb lead R wave or S wave≥ 20 mm S V1 or V2 ≥30 mm R V5 to R V6 ≥30 mm	3
ST-T abnormality (no digitalis therapy)	3
ST-T wave abnormality (digitalis therapy)	1
P terminal force in V1≥4mm/msec	3
QRS duration ≥ 0.095	1
Intrinsicoid deflection in V5 or V6 ≥50 m sec	1
Score >4 probable LVH, Score >5 definite LVH	

Paediatric Criteria for Left Ventricular Hypertrophy (Age-Related)

	Voltage (mm)				
	Age: 0-7d	Age: 7d -1y	Age: 1-3y	Age: 3-5y	Age: >5y
RV_6	>12	>23	>23	>25	>27
SV_1	>23	>18	>21	>22	>26
$SV1+R\,V_6$	>28	>35	>38	>42	>47

Based on Davignon et al. (48). Amplitudes are given in millimetres, where 1 mm = 0.1 mV.

Paediatric Criteria for Right Ventricular Hypertrophy (Age-Related)

Voltage (mm)					
	Age: 0-7d	Age: 7d -1y	Age: 1-3y	Age: 3-5y	Age: >5y
RV_1	>27	>22	>18	>18	>13
SV_5	>10	>10	>7	>6	>4
$SV1 + RV_6$	>37	>43	>30	>24	>17

■ STEPWISE CRITERIA FAVORING VENTRICULAR TACHYCARDIA

Brugada criteria	Miller criteria[4]
1. Absence of RS complex in all precordial leads VT	1. Initial R wave in aVR → VT
2. Longest R/S interval >100 msec in any precordial lead → VT	2. aVR with initial r or q > 40 msec in duration → VT
3. AV dissociation → VT	3. aVR with a notch on the descending limb of a negative-onset and predominantly negative QRS in aVR → VT
4. If RBBB morphology, monophasic R or qR in V1 → VT, R taller than R → VT, rS in V6→VT 5. If LBBB morphology, inital R>40 msec in duration → VT Slurred or notched S in V1 or V2 → VT	4. In aVR, mV of initial 40 msec divided by terminal 40 msec (v/v1≤1) → VT

REFERENCES

1. DeLuna AB. In: Text book of Clinical Electrocardiography. 1st Edition. Dordrecht: Martins Nijhoff; 1987.
2. Munuswamy, et al. Sensitivity and specificity of commonly used electrocardiographic criteria of left atrial enlargement determined by M mode Echocardiography. Am J Cardiology. 1984;53:829.
3. Hancok, et al. Standardization and interpretation of the ECG, part5, JACC. 2009;11:992-1002.
4. Verecki, et al. New algorithm using only lead avR for differential diagnosis of wide QRS tachycardia. Heart rhythm. 2008;5:89-98.

Index

Page numbers followed by *f* refer to figure and *t* refer to table

A

Abdomen 125
Acidosis, metabolic 5
Acne 193
Acquired arteriovenous fistula 94
Alveolar edema 240
American College of Rheumatology Criteria 182*t*
American Thoracic Society 1, 5
Anacrotic pulse 16
Anemia 5, 15, 91
Angina 7*t*, 8, 11, 112, 113, 119, 123, 160, 202
   caudal 8
   crescendo 8
   decubitus 7
   emotional 7
   mixed 7
   nocturnal 3, 7
   pectoris 63
   primary 7
   secondary 7
   silent 8
   warm-up 8
Angiogram 129, 217
   coronary 155
Ankylosing spondylitis 122
Annular patch 219
Annuloaortic ectasia 122, 181, 183
Anomalous pulmonary venous drainage 86
Anorexia 180
Anticoagulation 136, 148, 206
Anti-inflammatory drugs 106
Antiplatelet drugs 206
Antistreptolysin O 104
Anxiety 21
Aorta 15, 50, 59, 161
   coarctation of 14, 22, 59, 85, 91, 189
   dilatation of 112
   lesion, abdominal 182, 184
   overriding of 209

Aortic
   aneurysm 59, 185
   area 42
   closure 63
   component 52
   dissection 14
   ejection sound 53, 72, 73
   homograft 149
   impulse 50
   obstruction 180
   regurgitation 7, 15, 59, 80, 82, 111, 122, 128, 180, 181, 183, 185, 215
     severity of 81
   root
     disease 122
     surgery 118
   stenosis 6, 17, 110, 116*t*, 117*t*, 119, 142
     severe asymptomatic 117
     stenosis progression 118
     supravalvar 59
   valve 102, 116, 149
     disease 70, 112
     endocarditis 149
     lesion 119*t*
     replacement 118
Aortoarteritis 91, 178
Aortopulmonary collateral arteries 228
Arterial
   aneurysms 185
   blood pressure 23
   fistula, congenital coronary 92
   hypoxemia 3
   pulsations 31, 31*t*
   pulse 12, 123
     normal 14*f*
Arteriovenous fistula 15, 90
Artery
   dilatation, bronchial 91
   narrowing of 91
   palpation of 12
Arthralgia 180

Arthritis 98, 99, 106
  post-streptoccocal 99
  psoriatic 122
  viral 100
Aschoff nodule 101
Asthma 3, 4, 19
Atheletic heart 171*t*
Atresia, pulmonary 15, 91, 95
Atrial
  enlargement, left 164
  fibrillation 13, 36*f*, 38, 55, 56, 118, 131, 132*t*, 137, 143
  floor 32
  impulse 49
  myxoma 86, 134
  septal defect 38, 39, 76, 86
  systole 32
  tumor, right 38
Atrioventricular
  block 69
  ring 86
  valves 86
Atrium 237
Austin Flint murmur 88, 89, 89*t*, 134, 135*t*
Azithromycin 105

B

Baroreceptor mechanism 113
Benzathine penicillin G 105, 107
Bernheim's phenomenon 70
Bernheim's syndrome 35
Bicuspid aortic valve 85, 118
Bidirectional Glenn 221, 222
Bilateral diaphragmatic paralysis 3
Bioprosthetic valve 89
Bisferiens pulse 16, 17, 17*f*, 18*f*
  causes of 17*t*
Blackstone formula 220
Blalock Taussig, Waterston and Pott's shunt 90
Bland-White-Garland syndrome 94
Blood
  flow
    cephalization of 239
    pulmonary 91, 228, 239
  pressure 23, 26, 114
    systolic 128
  stream 124
  viscosity 193
Boot-shaped heart 215
Bridging therapy 154, 154*t*
Brokenbrough-Braunwald-Morrow sign 165
Bronchospasm 1
Brugada criteria 244

C

Calcium channel blockers 206
Carcinoma, bronchial 4
Carcinomatosis, lymphatic 5
Cardiac
  anomalies 211
  catheterization 91
  failure 66, 106
    chronic 4
    congestive 19, 117
  oxalosis 171
  tamponade 19
Cardiomyopathy
  arrhythmia induced 155
  hypertrophic 17, 158
  obstructive 160
  restrictive 38
Cardiovascular system 4
Carditis 99, 100, 101, 103*t*, 106
Carey-Coombs murmur 86, 134
Carotid
  artefact 32
  artery tenderness 181, 183
  pulse 161
Cephalosporin 105
Cerebral abscess 193
Cervical rib 14
Chamber hypertrophy 216
Chest
  pain 1, 7, 8, 132, 201
    atypical 7
    noncardiac 7
    typical 7
  tightness 1
  X-ray 115, 126, 135, 175, 186, 190, 215, 230, 235
Chordal rupture 102, 142, 145
Chorea 98, 99, 103
  treatment of 107
Cirrhosis 15, 91, 201-203, 218
Clindamycin 105
Cole-Cecil murmur 80
Complete heart block 13, 36, 38, 69, 88, 168

Consanguinity 192
Continuous murmur 90, 96, 194
Cor pulmonale 67
Coronary
  artery 180
    disease 69
    involvement 181
    lesion 184
  cameral fistula 91
  flow 123
  sinus 92
  stenosis 91
Corrigan's sign 124
Cruveilhier Blumgarten syndrome 91
Cyanosis 96, 193, 194, 218

D

Demusset's sign 124
Diabetes 112
  maternal 196, 210, 227
Dicrotic pulse 18, 18f
  causes of 18t
Digital erythema 218
Digoxin 204
Disopyramide 167
Distal brachiocephalic trunk lesion 182, 184
Dizziness 123
Dock's murmur 83
Down's syndrome 210
Dressler's grading 50
Drug therapy 167
Ductus arteriosus 15
Duroeziz's murmur 125
Dyslipedemia 112
Dyspnea 1, 2, 2f, 6, 8, 11, 113, 123, 131, 160, 201
  assessment, severity of 4
  causes of 4, 4t
  orthostatic 4
  sensation of 2

E

Ebstein's anomaly 56
Ectopic
  beats 56
  impulse 47
  pulsations 42
Edema
  interstitial 1
  laryngeal 5
  pedal 175

Eisenmenger syndrome 40, 201
Ejection
  click 72, 114
  sounds 72
  systolic murmur 114, 141, 214
Elbow pain 8
Emphysema 19, 56, 64
Endocarditis 145
  infective 122, 140, 142, 217
Epigastric impulse 50
Erythema
  marginatum 98, 99
  nodosum 180
European Society of Echo Guidelines 111t

F

Fallot's physiology 194
Fatigue 180
Fever 17, 98, 99, 180
Fibrosa 110
Flail mitral leaflet 57
Flow murmur 86
Fluroquinolones 105
Fluroscopy 151
Folic acid 192f
Fresh frozen plasma 155
Friedrich's ataxia 171
Friedrich's sign 37, 175

G

Gallavardian phenomenon 115
Gastrointestinal bleeding 113
Genetic disorders 210
Gerhard sign 125
Giant A wave 35
  causes of 35t
Gibson's murmur 91
Glenn shunt 222
Goldman specific activity scale 6t
Gonococcemia 100
Great arteries 59, 195

H

H wave 32
Haffman's variant 212
Headache 181

Heart
  beat, diastolic 53
  block 13
    Mobitz type 55
    second-degree 69
  disease
    congenital 4, 192, 198*t*, 201
    cyanotic 40, 40*t*, 91, 194, 197
    hypertensive 63, 171
    ischemic 140
    valvular 6
  failure 3, 6, 155, 194*t*, 241
    congestive 100, 143, 180, 181, 215
    severe biventricular 60
    symptoms 212
  lung transplant 206
  rate
    rapid 38
    slow 31*f*, 38
  size 235, 236
  sound 54, 58, 65, 66, 68, 69, 140, 141
    second 215
    soft first 56
  surgery, congenital 230
Hemangioma 91
Hemiplegia 181
Hemodynamics 110, 130, 165
  theory 189
Hemolysis 153
Hemoptysis 132, 201, 202
Hemostasis 193
Heparin 154
Hepatic venous hum 96
Hepatojugular reflux 33, 34
Hepatoma 91
Heterografts 148
Heyde syndrome 113
Hill's sign 125
Hoffman-Rigler sign 238
Hypercalcemia 112
Hyperdynamic apical cardiac impulse 46, 46*f*
Hyperinflation 1
Hyperkinetic
  heart syndrome 21
  pulse 14, 15, 15*f*
    causes of 15*t*
Hypernephroma 91
Hyperoxia test, role of 196
Hyperparathyroidism 112
Hypertension 27, 28, 56, 112, 180, 181, 183, 215
  acute 21
  severe 184
  pulmonary 11, 38, 60, 70, 91, 131, 155, 181, 200
  systemic 21, 59, 70
Hyperthyroidism 56
Hypertrophic obstructive cardiomyopathy 47
Hypertrophy
  asymmetric 159
  compensatory 110
  right ventricular 243
Hyperventilation, psychogenic 5
Hypoplasia 211
Hypotension, orthostatic 23

I

Infarction, pulmonary 201
Inflammatory bowel disease 181
Infundibular septum, malalignment of 209
Internal jugular vein 29
Interstitial pulmonary
  edema 240
  fibrosis 181
Ishikawa's criteria 181*t*

J

Jaccoud's arthritis 100
Jones criteria 98*t*, 99, 99*t*
Jordans hypothesis 131
Jugular venous
  pressure 33, 114
  pulse 29, 35*f*, 39*f*, 214
  tracing 36*f*-37*f*, 40*f*
  wave 40

K

Kawashima operation 221
Kerley's lines 239, 240*f*
Korotkoff sounds 24
Kussmaul's sign 38

L

Ladolfi's sign 124
Left ventricular
  hypertrophy 163, 209, 243
  outflow tract obstruction 16

Index

Leukemia, acute 100
Lev's disease 113
Lincoln sign 125
Lithium 196
Low dose dobutamine echo test 119
Lung
   disease, interstitial 4
   transplantation 206
Lutembacher syndrome 94

M

Malaise 180
Marfan's syndrome 122
Maron's classification 163
Mayne's sign 124
Meningococcemia 100
Mid-diastolic murmur 79, 83, 86*t*, 126, 134, 161
Mid-systolic accentuation 141
Milkmaid's grip 103
Miller criteria 244
Mitral regurgitation 6, 15, 60, 85, 140, 159, 164*t*
   severity, grading of 143*t*
Mitral stenosis 6, 36*f*, 55, 56, 76, 77, 83, 86, 127, 130, 134, 138, 139*f*
   severity of 77, 84, 130*t*, 134*t*
Mitral valve 54, 102, 149
   acute 102
   apparatus 130
   chronic 102
   obstruction 56
   prolapse 74, 140
   repair 145, 145*t*
   replacement 155
Monkeberg's sclerosis 22
Monoarthralgia 99
Morris index 136
Mucopolysaccharidosis 171
Muller's sign 124
Multiple peripheral pulmonary artery stenosis 95
Murmur 80, 119, 213
   diastolic 79, 80
   presystolic 135
   systolic 161
Muscles, papillary 159, 212
Musical diastolic murmur 81
Myectomy 168, 170*t*
Myer's classification 90
Myocardial
   disease 21
   fibrosis 159
   ischemia 1
      causes of 159
Myocarditis 101, 180, 181

N

Naito index 220
Nakata index 220
Nausea 181
Neck pain 123
New York Heart Association 4
   classification 5*t*
Night sweats 180
Nocturnal dyspnea, paroxysmal 3

O

Obesity 19, 64
Oliver-Cadarelli's sign 124
Orthodeoxia 3
Orthopnea 2
   causes of 3
Ortner syndrome 132
Osler's maneuver 22
Osteogenetic imperfecta 122
Oxygen saturation 204
Oxymetry 217
Pain 180
   abdominal 123
   pleuritic 180

P

Palpating distal artery 18
Paraesthesia 181
Paraplegia 181
Parasternal impulse 203
Parvus et tardus 114
Pasteur Rondot maneuver 33
Patent ductus arteriosus 17, 85, 90, 91
Pectus excavatum 61
Penicillin 105, 107
Pericardial
   autografts 148
   disease 21
   knock 77, 175
   tamponade 18
   valve 153
Pericarditis 181
   constrictive 19, 39, 47, 60, 174, 175

Perigraft seroma 221
Peripheral pulmonary stenosis 91
Phenylephrine 142
Phenylketonuria 227
   maternal 210
Plateau configuration 141
Platypnea 3
Pneumonia 4, 181
Pneumothorax 4
Polyarthralgia 98, 99
Polyarthritis 98, 99, 106
   migratory 100
Portal systemic shunt 91
Potts shunt 221
Propranalol 218
Prosthetic valve 147, 150*f*
   sounds 78
   stenosis 155
   thrombosis 151
Pseudohypertension 23
Pulmonary artery 50, 94, 95
   branch stenosis 95
   hypertension 239
   lesion 182, 184
   stenosis 231, 239
Pulmonary ejection
   click 73
   sound 53, 72
Pulmonary valve replacement 223
Pulmonary venous
   hypertension, grading of 240
Pulse
   trisection of 12
   volume of 21
Pulsus alternans 18, 19, 40*f*
   types of 19
Pulsus bigeminus 19, 19*f*
Pulsus paradoxus 19, 55, 161
   causes of 19*t*
Pulsus parvus et tardus 16, 16*f*

Q

Quadruple rhythm 66
Quincke's pulse 14
Quincke's sign 124

R

Regurgitation, pulmonary 82, 87, 222
Reiter's syndrome 122
Renal artery stenosis 91, 180
Renal failure 112
Respiratory
   distress syndrome, acute 5
   system 4
   tract infections, recurrent 214
Retinoic acid 196, 210, 227
Retinopathy 180, 184, 185
Rheumatic
   aortic regurgitation 128
   fever 97, 100, 107, 108*t*, 130
      acute 97, 101, 106
      prevention of 106
      recurrent 99
   heart disease 97, 98*t*, 140
   valvulitis 102*t*
Rheumatoid arthritis 122
Rib notching 190
   causes of 190
Romhilt-Estes point score system 243
Rosenbach sign 125
Rubella, maternal 196

S

Salicylates 106
Scoliosis 193
Seizures 181
Septal ablation 170
Septal defect
   large ventricular 76
   ventricular 15, 51, 85, 209
Seroma 220
Sherman sign 125
Shock 21
Shoulder pain 8
Shunts, types of 220
Sildenafil 204*f*
Sinus arrhythmia 13
Sinus of Valsalva 15, 91
   aneurysm 81, 85, 93
Skin 193
Sleep apnea 3
Soda bicarbonate 218
Somerville classification 230
Spongiosa 110
St Vitus dance 103
Stable angina 7
Stenosis 152
   pulmonary 35, 38, 60, 70, 74, 209

valvar 211
Sternal contact sign 238
Steroids 106
Straight back syndrome 61
Streptococcal antibody tests 104
Streptococcal infection 104
Streptokinase 151
Sulfadiazine 107
Sulfonamides 105
Surgery 91, 118, 144, 152, 219, 231
Sydenham's chorea 103
Syncope 1, 9, 9*t*, 10, 113, 119, 161, 166, 181, 202
Systolic sounds 72

T

Tachycardia 56, 66, 76
    junctional 38
    paroxysmal 36
    supraventricular 38
    ventricular 13, 38
Takayasu's arteritis 179
Takayasu's conference 180
Takayasu's disease 91
Takayasu's retinopathy 181
Tetracyclines 105
Tetralogy of Fallot 76, 209
Thalidomide 196
Thoracic aorta lesion 182, 184
Three-finger method 22
Throat culture 104
Thyrotoxicosis 15, 91
Tissue 147, 148
    valves 148, 149
Total anomalous pulmonary venous connection 96
Transcatheter aortic valve replacement 120, 155
Traube's sign 125
Trepopnea 4
Tricuspid
    atresia 35, 38, 76
    insufficiency 37*f*
    regurgitation 38, 39, 86, 155, 203
    murmur 175
    stenosis 35, 35*f*, 38, 76, 85, 88
    valve
        closure 54
        obstruction 56
Trimethadione 196, 210, 227
Trimethoprim 105
Truncus arteriosus 15, 95
Turner's syndrome 189

U

Upper limb 124
Uric acid 193

V

V wave 32, 37
Valproate 196
Valsalva maneuver 26, 26*f*, 27*f*
Valve
    closure, velocity of 55
    dysfunction 152
    involvement 101
    mobility of 55
    perforation 231
    types of 147
Valvular disease 21, 122
Valvular theory 65
Valvulitis 102*t*
Vascular theory 72
Veins
    pulmonary 195
    systemic 195
Velocardiofacial syndrome 211
Ventricular theory 65
Vomiting 181

W

Waterston shunt 221, 222
Whipples disease 100
White coat hypertension 23
Wide pulse pressure 124
Wiggle's scoring 163
Wilkins' echo score 138*t*
Wormian tongue 103